Current State of the Art in Spinal Cord Injury

Editor

JOHN HURLBERT

NEUROSURGERY
CLINICS OF NORTH AMERICA

www.neurosurgery.theclinics.com

Consulting Editors
RUSSELL R. LONSER
DANIEL K. RESNICK

July 2021 • Volume 32 • Number 3

ELSEVIER

1600 John F. Kennedy Boulevard • Suite 1800 • Philadelphia, Pennsylvania, 19103-2899

http://www.theclinics.com

NEUROSURGERY CLINICS OF NORTH AMERICA Volume 32, Number 3
July 2021 ISSN 1042-3680, ISBN-13: 978-0-323-81058-6

Editor: Stacy Eastman
Developmental Editor: Ann Gielou Posedio

Neurosurgery Clinics of North America (ISSN 1042-3680) is published quarterly by Elsevier Inc., 360 Park Avenue South, New York, NY 10010-1710. Months of issue are January, April, July, and October. Business and Editorial Offices: 1600 John F. Kennedy Blvd., Suite 1800, Philadelphia, PA 19103-2899. Customer Service Office: 11830 Westline Industrial Drive, St. Louis, MO 63146. Periodicals postage paid at New York, NY, and additional mailing offices. Subscription prices are $438.00 per year (US individuals), $1,013.00 per year (US institutions), $470.00 per year (Canadian individuals), $1,059.00 per year (Canadian institutions), $545.00 per year (international individuals), $1,059.00 per year (international institutions), $100.00 per year (US students), $255.00 per year (international students), and $100.00 per year (Canadian students). International air speed delivery is included in all *Clinics* subscription prices. All prices are subject to change without notice. **POSTMASTER:** Send address changes to *Neurosurgery Clinics of North America*, Elsevier Periodicals Customer Service, 11830 Westline Industrial Drive, St. Louis, MO 63146. **Customer Service: 1-800-654-2452 (US and Canada). From outside the US and Canada, call: 1-314-453-7041. Fax: 1-314-453-5170. E-mail: JournalsCustomerService-usa@elsevier.com (for print support) and journalsonlinesupport-usa@elsevier.com (for online support).**

Reprints. For copies of 100 or more, of articles in this publication, please contact the Commercial Reprints Department, Elsevier Inc., 360 Park Avenue South, New York, NY 10010-1710. Tel. 212-633-3874; Fax: 212-633-3820; E-mail: reprints@elsevier.com.

Neurosurgery Clinics of North America is covered in *MEDLINE/PubMed (Index Medicus), EMBASE/Excerpta Medica, and Current Contents/Clinical Medicine (CC/CM).*

Printed in the United States of America.

Contributors

CONSULTING EDITORS

RUSSELL R. LONSER, MD
Professor and Chair, Department of
Neurological Surgery, The Ohio State
University Wexner Medical Center, Columbus,
Ohio, USA

DANIEL K. RESNICK, MD, MS
Professor and Vice Chairman, Program
Director, Department of Neurosurgery,
University of Wisconsin-Madison School of
Medicine and Public Health, Madison,
Wisconsin, USA

EDITOR

JOHN HURLBERT, MD, PhD
Professor and Chief of Spinal Neurosurgery,
Department of Neurosurgery, University of
Arizona, Banner - University Medical Center
Tucson, Tucson, Arizona, USA

AUTHORS

MARK A. ANDERSON, PhD
Group Leader, Brain Mind Institute, Faculty of
Life Sciences, École Polytechnique Féderale
de Lausanne (EPFL), Leader, Neural Repair
Unit, NeuroRestore, Department of Clinical
Neuroscience, Lausanne University Hospital
(CHUV) and University of Lausanne (UNIL),
Lausanne, Switzerland

MAURICIO J. AVILA, MD
Chief Resident, Department of Neurosurgery,
University of Arizona, Banner - University
Medical Center Tucson, Tucson, Arizona, USA

MATTHEW D. BUDDE, PhD
Department of Neurosurgery, Medical College
of Wisconsin, Wauwatosa, Wisconsin, USA;
Clement J Zablocki Veteran's Affairs Medical
Center, Milwaukee, Wisconsin, USA

JOHN F. BURKE, MD, PhD
Department of Neurological Surgery, University
of California, San Francisco, San Francisco,
California, USA

IAHN CAJIGAS, MD, PhD
Chief Resident, Department of Neurosurgery,
University of Miami, Miami, Florida, USA

JENS R. CHAPMAN, MD
Department of Neurosurgery, Swedish
Neuroscience Institute, Seattle, Washington,
USA

ANDREW T. DAILEY, MD
Department of Neurosurgery, Clinical
Neurosciences Center, University of Utah, Salt
Lake City, Utah, USA

SANJAY S. DHALL, MD
Department of Neurological Surgery, University
of California, San Francisco, San Francisco,
California, USA

MICHAEL G. FEHLINGS, MD, PhD
Division of Neurosurgery, Department of
Surgery, University of Toronto, Division of
Neurosurgery, Krembil Neuroscience Centre,
Toronto Western Hospital, University Health
Network, Toronto, Ontario, Canada

LAUREEN D. HACHEM, MD
Division of Neurosurgery, Department of Surgery, University of Toronto, Division of Neurosurgery, Krembil Neuroscience Centre, Toronto Western Hospital, University Health Network, Toronto, Ontario, Canada

ALEXANDER F. HADDAD, BS
Department of Neurological Surgery, University of California, San Francisco, San Francisco, California, USA

JOHN HURLBERT, MD, PhD
Professor and Chief of Spinal Neurosurgery, Department of Neurosurgery, University of Arizona, Banner - University Medical Center Tucson, Tucson, Arizona, USA

ALLAN D. LEVI, MD, PhD
Professor and Chairman, Department of Neurological Surgery, University of Miami Miller School of Medicine, Lois Pope Life Center, Miami, Florida, USA

NIKOLAY L. MARTIROSYAN, MD, PhD
Department of Neurosurgery, Allen Memorial Hospital, UnityPoint Clinic, Waterloo, Iowa, USA

BRIANA P. MEYER, BS
Departments of Neurosurgery, and Biophysics, Medical College of Wisconsin, Wauwatosa, Wisconsin, USA

MARIOS C. PAPADOPOULOS, MD, FRCS(SN)
Professor, Department of Neurosurgery, Atkinson Morley Wing, St. George's Hospital NHS Foundation Trust, London, United Kingdom

WYATT L. RAMEY, MD
Department of Neurosurgery, Banner - University Medical Center Tucson, Tucson, Arizona, USA

SAMIRA SAADOUN, PhD
Senior Lecturer in Neuroscience, Academic Neurosurgery Unit, St. George's, University of London, London, United Kingdom

SAMAN SHABANI, MD
Department of Neurosurgery, Medical College of Wisconsin, Wauwatosa, Wisconsin, USA

CHARLES H. TATOR, OC, MD, PhD, FRCSC, FACS
Professor of Neurosurgery, University of Toronto, and Krembil Brain Institute, Toronto Western Hospital, Founder, ThinkFirst Canada and Parachute Canada, Director, Tator SCI Laboratory, Krembil Brain Institute, Toronto Western Hospital, University Health Network, Toronto, Ontario, Canada

ADITYA VEDANTAM, MD
Minimally Invasive and Complex Spine Fellow, Department of Neurological Surgery, University of Miami Miller School of Medicine, Lois Pope Life Center, Miami, Florida, USA

MARJORIE C. WANG, MD, MPH
Department of Neurosurgery, Medical College of Wisconsin, Wauwatosa, Wisconsin, USA

CHRISTOPHER WILKERSON, MD
Department of Neurosurgery, Clinical Neurosciences Center, University of Utah, Salt Lake City, Utah, USA

Contents

Basics of SCI

Laureen D. Hachem and Michael G. Fehlings

> Spinal cord injury (SCI) triggers a complex cascade of molecular and cellular events that leads to progressive cell loss and tissue damage. In this review, the authors outline the temporal profile of SCI pathogenesis, focusing on key mediators of the secondary injury, and highlight cutting edge insights on the alterations in neural circuits that largely define the chronic injury environment. They bridge these important basic science concepts with clinical implications for informing novel experimental therapies. Furthermore, emerging concepts in the study of SCI pathogenesis that are transforming fundamental research into innovative clinical treatment paradigms are outlined.

Alexander F. Haddad, John F. Burke, and Sanjay S. Dhall

> The natural history of spinal cord injury is in a state of flux. Our knowledge about the prevalence, epidemiology, and natural history spinal cord injury is in evolution. In this article, we summarize these considerations to provide a state-of-the-art synopsis of the neurologic outcomes of this condition.

Saman Shabani, Briana P. Meyer, Matthew D. Budde, and Marjorie C. Wang

> In the evaluation of spinal trauma, diagnostic imaging is of paramount importance. Computed tomography (CT), flexion/extension radiographs, and MRI are complementary modalities. CT is typically obtained in the initial setting of spinal trauma and provides detailed information about osseous structures. MRI provides detailed information about structural injury to the spinal cord. Diffusion tensor imaging provides microstructural information about the integrity of the axons and myelin sheaths, but its clinical use is limited. Novel imaging techniques may be better suited for the acute clinical setting and are under development for potential future clinical use.

Wyatt L. Ramey and Jens R. Chapman

> Spinal cord injury (SCI) remains a challenging disease in terms of surgical decision-making and improving neurologic outcome. As we have now entered a new era founded on routine "big data" capture, more advanced and meaningful yet simplified SCI classification systems and outcome measurement tools would be helpful to

determine the efficacy of potential therapeutics in future clinical trials and registries. The proposed classification herein focuses on gross sensorimotor, sacral function below the injured level via an easy-to-use scoring system yielding grades 1 to 4 of injury severity. Such an optimized SCI scoring system would enhance real-time analytics and offer superior outcomes modeling.

neuroprotective strategy that can be combined with other therapies. Systemic hypothermia affects several processes at the cellular level to reduce metabolic activity, oxidative stress, and apoptotic neuronal cell death. Modest systemic hypothermia has been shown to be safe and feasible in the acute phase after cervical spinal cord injury. These data have provided the impetus for an active multicenter randomized controlled trial for modest systemic hypothermia in acute cervical spinal cord injury.

NEUROSURGERY CLINICS OF NORTH AMERICA

SERIES OF RELATED INTEREST

Neurologic Clinics
https://www.neurologic.theclinics.com/
Neuroimaging Clinics
https://www.neuroimaging.theclinics.com/

THE CLINICS ARE AVAILABLE ONLINE!
Access your subscription at:
www.theclinics.com

Preface

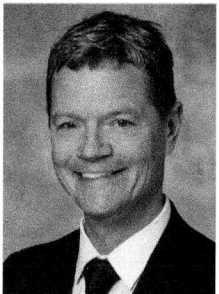

John Hurlbert, MD, PhD
Editor

This issue of *Neurosurgery Clinics of North America* focuses on one of the most long-lasting, life-altering conditions known to our specialty: spinal cord injury (SCI). Since the inaugural issue in 1990, *Neurosurgery Clinics of North America* has been publishing quarterly state-of-the-art updates intended to keep students, researchers, and surgeons on the cutting edge of information specific to our discipline. In acknowledging this 30-year legacy, it is fitting we recognize and dedicate this issue to a world-renowned student, researcher, and clinical master, who has dedicated his career to the pursuit of Spinal Cord Injury, and continues to leave a growing legacy in his footsteps, Dr Charles Haskell Tator (**Fig. 1**).

Born and raised in Toronto, Dr Tator earned his MD from the University of Toronto in 1961 and followed shortly thereafter with a PhD in Neuropathology. He finished his Neurosurgical Residency training at the University of Toronto in 1969 and became one of the first dedicated clinician-scientists in Neurosurgery, starting his basic science SCI laboratory at Sunnybrook Health Sciences Center in 1971. This lab, now located at Toronto Western Hospital, remains productive today with Dr Tator active at the helm. The lab has been well funded from multiple sources and has been awarded over $10M in the past 15 years alone.

Over this 50-year legacy, Dr Tator and his lab have produced more than four hundred peer-reviewed publications, trained 49 research fellows, and played an important founding role in our current understanding of key translational aspects of the pathobiology and treatment of SCI. Among the many seminal research contributions made by Dr Tator, perhaps most important relates to defining the critical aspects of vascular disruption as a key driver of secondary injury. Dr Tator is a Fellow of both the Royal College of Physicians and Surgeons of Canada and the American College of Surgeons; he has been inducted into the Canadian Sports Hall of Fame and is an Officer of the Order of Canada.

Dr Charles ("Husky") Tator has shown those of us lucky enough to have trained with him that through painstaking and careful analysis of both basic science and clinical data we can begin to move the needle forward and develop a deeper understanding and meaningful treatments for our SCI patients. We are honored to have been awakened and inspired by Dr Tator's mentorship and are forever grateful for the wisdom he has imparted. Without a doubt, he has become a surrogate father for us all… the highest compliment possible.

This issue of *Neurosurgery Clinics of North America* provides the reader with an eyes-wide-open view of where we're headed in the treatment

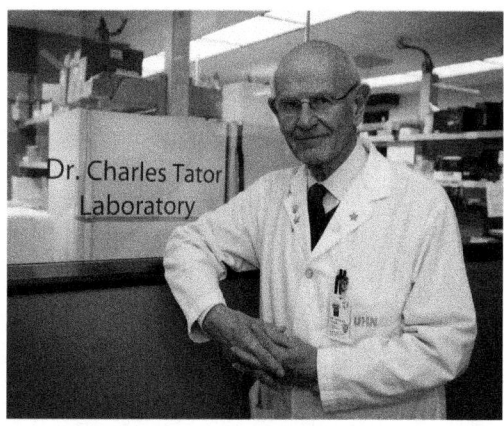

Fig. 1. Dr. Tator and his Spinal Cord Injury laboratory

Neurosurg Clin N Am 32 (2021) ix–x
https://doi.org/10.1016/j.nec.2021.04.002
1042-3680/21/© 2021 Published by Elsevier Inc.

of acute SCI, framed in the context of where we've come from and where we are now. Dr Tator kindly kicks the issue off with a perspective adding the most important element of all, the human element. To the readership of *Neurosurgery Clinics of North America*, sit back and enjoy. To Dr Tator, "thank you" doesn't even begin to express the debt owed. But on behalf of a grateful profession, and from every Neurosurgeon around the world... this one's for you.

John Hurlbert, MD, PhD
Department of Neurosurgery
Banner University Medical Center
PO Box 245070
1501 North Campbell Avenue, Room 4303
Tucson, AZ 85724-5070, USA

Allan D. Levi, MD, PhD (contributor)
Department of Neurological Surgery
University of Miami Miller School of Medicine
Lois Pope Life Center
1095 Northwest 14th Terrace, Suite 2-24
Miami, FL 33136, USA

Michael G. Fehlings, MD, PhD (contributor)
Division of Neurosurgery
Department of Surgery
University of Toronto
Division of Neurosurgery
Toronto Western Hospital
University Health Network
Toronto, ON, Canada

E-mail address:
rjhurlbert@email.arizona.edu

Introduction
Spinal Cord Injury: Journey of Discovery

I am grateful to John Hurlbert, Russ Lonser, and Dan Resnick for asking me to participate in this important issue on spinal cord injury (SCI). John and I have known each other for a long time. He was a superb research fellow in my SCI lab, and an excellent resident on my neurosurgical service. I am honored to write this introductory article, and my goal is to portray for readers some of the excitement I experienced and the important milestones in SCI management and research that I was privileged to witness. So much has happened in this journey of discovery that I had the good fortune to witness.

CLINICAL MANAGEMENT OF SPINAL CORD INJURY AND MY BEGINNING IN THE SPINAL CORD INJURY FIELD

By the time this issue is published, it will be a half century since I published my first SCI paper.[1] My interest in SCI predated that by about 10 years and occurred when I was a junior intern at the Toronto General Hospital assigned to the operating room to assist a master surgeon. This surgeon was trained when the twentieth century began, and there were no distinctions between surgical specialties. A surgeon could remove an appendix one day, do a mitral valvotomy the next, and then a spinal cord tumor. Also, this surgeon was one of the few who had a laboratory in which he told me he was researching removal of a vertebra to shorten the spinal column and relieve tension at the site of SCI "to get paralyzed people walking again." In the month of my assignment, I assisted him on one of these "vertebrectomy" operations on a patient in which the surgeon meticulously opened the dura and exposed the damaged, scarred, and atrophic spinal cord. Later that month, I was assigned to do the admission history and physical examination on another of this surgeon's patients who was scheduled for this operation the next day. The amazing thing about this C5-6 quadriplegic patient in his 20s was that *he could walk* prior to the operation, and I saw it myself. It was the first time I witnessed "crutch walking." Postoperatively he could still walk. However, it was revealed during an enquiry several years later that an actual vertebrectomy had not been performed in this patient, or in the others who were also supposed to have had the operation. The vertebrectomy had only been accomplished in rabbits in this surgeon's lab, as I learned later when I did a literature review. This surreal experience and controversy had an effect on me and was one of the reasons I developed a basic science laboratory in SCI in 1970, one of the first in Canada. Indeed, I was permanently hooked on SCI as something that needed fixing.

Also, indelibly imprinted on my brain was my exposure to Harry Botterell, the chief of Neurosurgery in Toronto after I decided that was the field for me. I was the last resident he accepted into the program before he left for Queens University in Kingston, Ontario to be their new Dean of Medicine. Botterell was a giant physically and mentally. Also, as a junior intern I watched him do the first "Cloward procedure" in Canada. He had made a huge contribution to the SCI field during the second World War as a surgeon treating SCI war victims at the military hospital in Basingstoke, England. Canadian war-wounded with SCI were then repatriated to Christie Street Hospital, then to Lyndhurst Lodge, both in Toronto, and then to Sunnybrook Hospital, a veteran's hospital in Toronto. During neurosurgical training in Toronto, I completed a PhD (I think the first surgeon in Canada to do an "infolded" PhD during Neurosurgical training). When training was over in 1969, I was told by my next Chief, Tom Morley, "You are going to be the first University of Toronto full-time neurosurgeon at Sunnybrook," which had just been bought by the University. At Sunnybrook, I helped look after all the veterans with SCI who were domiciled there and who had an amazing array of spinal problems for me to deal with dating from the war, including unstable spinal fracture-dislocations, intractable pain, posttraumatic and post-Thorotrast (myelogram contrast) syringomyelia, and ensuing arachnoiditis. Thus, being appointed to Sunnybrook sealed my career as a committed SCI practitioner and researcher.

GRADING OF SPINAL CORD INJURY SEVERITY, SCORING OF SPINAL CORD INJURY RECOVERY, AND BIOMARKERS

Grading and scoring of SCI have been major pursuits and continue to be important endeavors for SCI clinicians and researchers, as exemplified in this issue. I observed remarkable progress in the

1042-3680/21/© 2021 Published by Elsevier Inc.

past 50 years, which has improved quality control in both clinical care and clinical trials. In the early 1960s, all we had was "complete and incomplete, and motor and sensory" to characterize the injury. The Frankel scale was a leap forward, soon to be replaced by the ASIA grading and scoring system. I participated in this work, first as the author of a new system of grading and scoring,[2] and then as a Committee Member on the very useful ASIA and international systems to which I contributed the method to define the difference between grades C and D. The Japanese Orthopedic Association scale came along and has endured, as have the FIM and Israeli SCIM systems for gauging rehabilitation results. These systems have all maintained their usefulness. However, we need improved precision for gauging prognosis and treatment effects. This should be achievable with biomarkers in biofluids, imaging, or some other modality. Years ago, we had hoped that electrophysiologic measures of motor and sensory conduction in the spinal cord would be an important gauge of the extent of injury and the prognosis. I spent about 25 years trying to make this happen, but unfortunately there was no benefit, although it is still useful for early warning in the operating room. There is still hope for MRI, and I am pleased that Michael Fehlings, another neurosurgeon I supervised as a researcher and then as a resident, remains in pursuit of this goal.[3] Michael is the senior author of the lead article in this issue of *Neurosurgery Clinics of North America*, beautifully summarizing the pathophysiology of SCI.

MODELING THE INJURY

When I began at Sunnybrook, my first basic science lab was 10 kilometers away at the Banting Institute in Toronto. Within a few years, the lab moved to the Medical Sciences Building on the University of Toronto main campus where I was able to house nonhuman primates for SCI research. I invented an inflatable circumferential cuff to deliver the injury, and although we could measure the force *in* the cuff, we could not measure the force *between* the cuff and adjacent cord. It was then that I wrote my first papers on experimental SCI.[1,4] In fact, I got so hooked on SCI research that I was advised by Tom Morley to focus on this and give up experimental brain tumor research, which I had carried over from my PhD days.

EARLY CARE AND INTENSIVE CARE FOR SPINAL CORD INJURY

In the early 1970s, Sunnybrook Hospital decided that its future was in being a trauma center, indeed Canada's first dedicated trauma center, and I was integral to the planning and execution of that development because I was the only neurosurgeon for miles around. So, I began plenty of on-the-job learning about acute SCI, especially nights and weekends. I learned how to line vertebrae up with halos and how to reduce and fuse fracture-dislocations operatively. Early liaison with orthopedic surgeons was essential. I was not a speedy surgeon, but I became obsessed with speed of management of SCI, because of what I saw clinically and what I learned in my lab: the sooner we got the pressure off the cord, the better the outcome. Thus, I advocated for patient referral as soon as possible after injury, but soon realized it required the cooperation of many. There was huge systemic inertia and ambivalence about the necessity for early treatment of SCI, even among my colleagues, many of whom were superb clinicians. Socialized medicine had arrived in Ontario in the 1960s, so no changes of the magnitude I was recommending could be accomplished without the buy-in of the Ministry of Health of Ontario, which, for example, directed the ambulance services. Harry Botterell went into action and strongly supported the plan I presented to him for developing one of the first Acute Spinal Cord Injury Units in the world. He was very influential with the Ministry of Health, and his admirable war work in the SCI field made him the strongest advocate for change. It was a done deal. To be sure, there was scoffing from some of the "old guard" who had a very nihilistic approach to acute SCI and were influenced by lots of SCI gurus worldwide, including Sir Ludwig Guttman in Britain, Sir George Bedbrook in Australia, and several US giants like Donald Munro in Boston, who regarded surgical treatment of acute SCI as dangerous to the spinal cord and a threat to the life of the SCI patient. They "knew" that all was over as soon as the injury happened, and all you could do was to make sure you did no additional harm. In contrast, during the first few years of our Acute SCI Unit, we showed that early surgical treatment was indeed beneficial for cord recovery in comparison with what had been achieved previously, and that it could be done safely.[5,6] We also showed that in experimental animals the same was true: early decompression improved neurologic recovery, first in monkeys[4] and later in rats.[7] To do the latter, we devised the first small animal model of acute SCI with a modified aneurysm clip[8] with which we could vary *both* the force and the duration of compression of the rat spinal cord, which we had been unable to do with the cuff in monkeys. These laboratory successes encouraged me to initiate the Surgical Treatment of Acute Spinal Cord Injury Study (STASCIS) project in SCI patients to examine whether early surgical decompression was beneficial. At the time, the American Association of Neurological Surgeons and Congress of Neurological Surgeons Joint Section on Neurotrauma was instrumental in supporting these clinical trials. We did some pilot studies that were encouraging[9] and then planned a large-scale randomized controlled trial of early surgical decompression for patients in North America.[10] Unfortunately, funding for the STASCIS randomized trial was rejected by National Institutes of Health (NIH). However, ultimately, we did it anyway, and proved the value and safety of early surgical decompression, although by that time there was no longer equipoise about early treatment, and so it could not be a randomized design. Michael Fehlings[11] led the final trial that showed the value of early decompression of the spinal cord after SCI in patients.

UNRAVELLING THE PATHOPHYSIOLOGY OF SPINAL CORD INJURY AND EFFORTS TO PROVIDE NEUROPROTECTION

I was drawn into the world of trying to discover what was really going on inside the injured spinal cord. We had witnessed the remarkable improvements afforded by safe, early surgery, and that it was better than the old technique of no surgery, waiting instead for eventual stability after months of log-rolling bed-bound patients while bone healed, hoping they did not succumb to pressure sores, urinary tract infections, and pulmonary emboli. However, we still needed better treatments than steroids to combat the ravages of the hostile pathophysiology of SCI. There was a cadre of investigators spanning many countries that had developed from the 1960s to the 1980s or so, and the driving forces were the International Medical Society of Paraplegia and the International Neurotrauma Society, which had amazing meetings of those investigators for traumatic brain injury and SCI. There were giants and pioneers like Graham Teasdale, Wise Young, Jewell Osterholm, Paul Reier, and others, who were making great discoveries at the bench. Jewell's "noradrenaline theory" went around the world with lots of labs, including my own, racing to the battle with ways to counteract, for example, the impoverished blood flow to marginally perfused penumbra tissue. This group identified spectacular ionic fluxes into and out of injured tissue, leaving behind a glutamate storm cloud, which somehow induced NMDA receptors to let in too much calcium, which then wrecked nervous tissue. The experts predicted, for example, that this could be counteracted by calcium channel blockers. By this time, my SCI

lab had moved to the Toronto Western Hospital, and we had a great time, where stars like Michael Fehlings, John Hurlbert, and Michael Tymianski could apply their brilliance. It was a time when research funding agencies developed in many countries often at the urging of spectacular personalities like Christopher Reeve and Nick Buoniconti in the United States, Rick Hansen and Barbara Turnbull in Canada, and Stuart Yesner in the United Kingdom and Australia, who strongly supported SCI research through their public appeals, personal experiences, and pleadings. As well, government agencies like NIH in the United States and Canadian Institutes of Health Research (CIHR) in Canada got on the bandwagon to fund SCI research, and even clinical trials like NASCIS. We did not realize it at the time, but it was probably the "hay-day" for funding bench-to-bedside SCI research, because it has been downhill for funding ever since.

As noted above, when I approached NIH to fund the STASCIS surgical trial, the answer was "no." What emerged from all this was a clear understanding about how formidable the enemy SCI is. Not only was there electrolyte imbalance, edema, ischemia, vasospasm, infarction, inflammation, astrocytic scars, and CSPG barriers but also there were major inhibitors of regeneration like Nogo and RGMa lurking around ground zero, the injury site. This field is still highly promising as shown by work in my lab during the past 5 years, led by Andrea Mothe. Our positive results in restoring some locomotion and bladder function in rats with an anti-RGMa antibody was a significant driver for the current clinical trial of anti-RGMa antibody in patients with cervical cord SCI.[12,13] The beneficial effect of hypothermia on all of these secondary injury mechanisms remains an exciting avenue of research spearheaded by another of my superstar neurosurgery residents, Allan Levi. Allan has contributed a superb update on this promising therapy and ongoing work at the Miami project in his article in this issue.

And so, my message to current and budding SCI investigators is that there is still a great need for continuing discoveries in this area. Please join the swim! Here is the challenge: solve this mystery! Discover which vasospastic agent released at the lesion epicenter and in the penumbra after SCI is the main culprit for posttraumatic ischemia and infarction of the injured spinal cord![14]

THE EXCITEMENT OF STEM CELLS FOR REGENERATING THE INJURED SPINAL CORD

In 1996, Canadian investigators announced that the adult mammalian spinal cord contains stem cells that can be stimulated to divide and generate new neurons and glial cells.[15] I remember thinking at the time that this could be the explanation for an observation I had made many years before in rat clip impact-compression injury: the ependymal cells lining the central canal at both rostral and caudal edges of the necrotic injury epicenter were piled up and multilayered in contrast to the usual single layer of cells, and that even the central canal could be duplicated. Yes, ependymal region stem cells accounted for these events as we and others subsequently proved: ependymal cells proliferate in response to trauma. We showed that a small percentage of ependymal cells lining the central canal were in fact multipotential stem cells and could generate neurons, astrocytes, and oligodendroglial cells. Indeed, we could generate more of them by several strategies, including the administration of growth factors. However, when we tried to exploit their regenerative potential for improving function after SCI, the functional effect on activities such as locomotion was disappointing.[16,17] Nevertheless, manipulation of endogenous stem cells is still a viable strategy. Indeed, we are still at it in my lab more than 20 years later based on a recent discovery made by Laureen Hachem, now a neurosurgical resident and graduate student. She discovered that these cells have a paradoxical response to glutamate and that their survival and proliferation are *enhanced* in vitro by glutamate excess.[18]

The other stem cell strategy is transplantation of exogenous stem cells into the injured spinal cord to regenerate lost tissue. Indeed, almost all current stem cell activity in SCI in the laboratory and in patients now involves transplantation of various types of stem/progenitor cells. For transplantation, I favor neural stem cells, mainly those derived from induced pluripotential cells to avoid the necessity for long-term, concomitant immunosuppression. It is quite thrilling that there have been at least 3 trials of the use of transplanted stem cells in patients with SCI, but final long-term results are not available. In my view, the trials have been well done and have been safe. They have been very expensive, and all were initiated, organized, and paid for by private companies. The technology of cell preparation, transport, storage, and safe transplantation into the injured cord seems to have worked very well. However, study curtailment was often necessary for financial reasons. Sadly, there were no government rescues, and no government funding of any stem cell trials in human SCI in any country. Long-term follow-up is essential for assessment of effectiveness, complications, and safety and is still pending, but perhaps that is acceptable because of the slowness of regeneration in the human central nervous system.

THE IMAGING REVOLUTION IN SPINAL CORD INJURY

In my career, the evolution of imaging for SCI has progressed from plain radiographs, to safe myelography, computed tomography (CT), and then to MRI and has been accompanied by great joy on the part of both patients and practitioners. When I began, we were unable to visualize the spinal cord except in the "mind's eye" or by shadows, and then came actual visualization with CT and MRI. MRI for SCI was truly revolutionary, not so much experimentally, but certainly for clinical management, especially for incomplete injuries, such as the central cord syndrome. Also, MRI presented us with amazing clinical evidence of what we had observed in experimental studies in animals and in infrequent autopsies in patients soon after SCI, that there is extensive anteroposterior and rostrocaudal extent and spread of the SCI lesion. As noted above, there is still reasonable hope that MRI will ultimately be a reliable biomarker and provide reliable prognostic information.[3] Dr Marjorie Wang and her colleagues have provided a very nice overview of this in their article in this issue.

THE MULTIDISCIPLINARY NATURE OF THE SPINAL CORD INJURY FIELD, AND THE NEED FOR LEADERSHIP AND CONCENTRATION

Similar to most other areas in medicine, management of SCI patients requires a multidisciplinary team, and this has become even more evident as knowledge about the pathophysiology of SCI has accumulated. SCI affects so many functions that a multidisciplinary team is essential, and this was recognized from the onset of organized care more than 100 years ago. The care journey of an SCI patient requires a "village" to do the job properly from the scene of injury through rehabilitation and beyond, including saying farewell to those who don't survive. The list of health care professionals often required is monumental to give the patient the "best shot" at recovering: social worker, physiotherapist, occupational therapist, speech therapist, and respiratory therapist; and in medical disciplines, the following may all be required: intensivist, neurosurgeon, orthopedic surgeon, physiatrist, urologist, psychiatrist, neuroradiologist, and others. The team is supposed to "play nicely in the sandbox," and in general, this has happened during the span of my career, but not always. Leadership and nurturing are required. Who the leaders are varies from country to country, often based on tradition rather than skills and talent. However, there has been enormous progress with more gains expected. Personally, it has been a pleasure to interact with an array of practitioners from other disciplines, and I am thinking of giants like John DiTunno in Rehab Medicine and Sukhvinder Kalsi Ryan in physiotherapy. The need for a multidisciplinary team, working with specialized diagnostic and treatment equipment, is compounded by the small number of SCI cases in a given location. Thus, it is imperative to regionalize SCI care to achieve optimal results. The high cost of excellent care is the driving force. Many years ago, we demonstrated cost savings from regionalized SCI care, but unfortunately, the results were not published. In many countries, economics has driven the development of regionalized centers for acute and rehabilitation SCI care, sometimes in the same location, but generally separate.

SUPPORT FOR SPINAL CORD INJURY RESEARCH

Major progress has been made during the past 50 years in the understanding and management of SCI, largely due to the inventiveness of a multitude of SCI researchers and clinicians aided by an amazing amount of goodwill and philanthropy on the part of governments and private foundations in many countries. During this time, great public institutions like the American NIH and Canadian CIHR began providing funds for SCI research as well as great feedback to investigators seeking to do clinical and basic science SCI research. Also, nongovernment organizations and foundations came forward with significant funding for SCI research. In the United Kingdom, the International Spinal Research Trust founded by Stewart Yesner provided funds to researchers in many countries, including me. In the United States and Canada, there were many SCI funders, including the Christopher Reeve Foundation, Craig H. Neilsen Foundation, Morton Cure Paralysis Fund, Rick Hansen Man in Motion Foundation, and the Barbara Turnbull Foundation. In Europe, Wings for Life Spinal Cord Research Foundation and the International Institute for Research in Paraplegia have been noteworthy funders. Many philanthropic efforts in SCI were started or enhanced by SCI patients themselves, including Christopher Reeve, Stewart Yesner, Rick Hansen, Barbara Turnbull, Peter Morton, Craig Neilson, and others. SCI research funding seemed to reach its zenith toward the end of the last century. Unfortunately, in the last 20 years in many countries, both governmental and nongovernmental sources of funding for clinical and basic science SCI research have gradually diminished. For example, the NIH declined to fund the STASCIS trial of early decompression in the late 1990s, and indeed, the last *major* SCI clinical trial funded by NIH was probably the NASCIS trial of methylprednisolone in the 1980s. Funding for fundamental SCI research has also dwindled from the governmental and private agencies listed above, such as ISRT in the United Kingdom, Christopher Reeve in the United States, and Rick Hansen in Canada, which have all ceased to offer their annual open funding awards competitions. Another negative indicator is that almost all the recent clinical trials in SCI, whether drug trials like Cethrin or Riluzole or stem cell trials, have mostly been company-initiated and company-funded trials. Governments now put a disproportionate percentage of their resources into the larger disease entities at the expense of lower incidence conditions like SCI. One of the world's exceptions, of course, is the US military, which continues to fund an array of SCI research. The overall funding shortfall and maldistribution are especially unfortunate for current and future SCI sufferers, and also those interested in performing SCI research who may be keen to pursue this less "popular" condition as I was, but are forced to join the "biggies" who have more resources.

EPIDEMIOLOGY AND PREVENTION OF SPINAL CORD INJURY

There have always been remarkable disparities among countries in the incidence of SCI, and often the differences relate to the number of motor vehicles in a country or the presence of hazardous workplaces. Motor vehicle crashes, sports, and recreation have predominated in many countries in terms of risk, while work and violence (including domestic violence) have been less common. There has always been a large male preponderance in the incidence of SCI, often a 5:1 male to female ratio.[19] In most mechanisms of injury except falls, a higher incidence has been in young adults, but as injury prevention efforts increase with respect to making sports safer, including safer recreational activities such as diving, SCI in young adults is declining. With more people living longer, falls among the elderly are shifting the demographics of SCI toward an older age group and also tending to even the male to female ratio.[20,21] This has also been nicely reviewed in John Hurlbert's contribution to this issue on central cord syndrome.

Examples of effective prevention efforts in SCI include a wide range of activities in sports and recreation, such as a reduction in broken necks in hockey due to greater awareness and stiffer penalties against hitting from behind, and the Head and spinal immobilization system in motorsport racing. In the case of prevention of SCI in motor vehicle crashes, there is now widespread installation and use of seat belts and airbags in all motor vehicles. If occupants remain inside during a crash, the incidence of SCI declines. In the work environment, improved training and safety harnesses have been effective. Finally, one of the most common mechanisms of SCI in the elderly, falls at home, is being addressed by fall-prevention programs focused on seniors. Prevention of SCI remains our most effective means of treating this catastrophic injury, even now in the twenty-first century.

SUMMARY

Thank you to the readership for indulging me in the opportunity to reminisce and comment about the field of SCI in general and about my personal experiences. It has been a great thrill to be involved, and I hope the future will continue to provide the same excitement to the readers and increased benefits to those injured who live with the consequences of SCI.

Charles H. Tator, OC, MD, PhD, FRCSC, FACS
Division of Neurosurgery
Toronto Western Hospital
399 Bathurst Street, Suite 4W-422
Toronto, ON M5T 2S8, Canada

E-mail address:
charles.tator@uhn.ca

REFERENCES

1. Tator CH. Experimental circumferential compression injury of primate spinal cord. Proc Veterans Adm Spinal Cord Inj Conf 1971;18:2–5.
2. Tator CH, Rowed DW, Schwartz ML. Sunnybrook cord injury scales for assessing neurological injury and recovery. In: Tator CH, editor. Early management of acute spinal cord injury. New York: Raven Press; 1982.
3. Freund P, Seif M, Weiskopf N, et al. MRI in traumatic spinal cord injury: from clinical assessment to neuroimaging biomarkers. Lancet Neurol 2019; 18(12):1123–35.
4. Tator CH. Acute spinal cord injury in primates produced by an inflatable extradural cuff. Can J Surg 1973;16(3):222–31.
5. Tator CH, Edmonds VE. Acute spinal cord injury: analysis of epidemiologic factors. Can J Surg 1979;22(6):575–8.
6. Tator CH, Rowed DW. Current concepts in the immediate management of acute spinal cord injuries. Can Med Assoc J 1979;121(11):1453–64.
7. Dolan EJ, Tator CH, Endrenyi L. The value of decompression for acute experimental spinal cord compression injury. J Neurosurg 1980;53(6):749–55.
8. Rivlin AS, Tator CH. Effect of duration of acute spinal cord compression in a new acute cord injury model in the rat. Surg Neurol 1978;10(1):38–43.
9. Ng WP, Fehlings MG, Cuddy B, et al. Surgical treatment for acute spinal cord injury study pilot study #2: evaluation of protocol for decompressive surgery within 8 hours of injury. Neurosurg Focus 1999;6(1):e3.
10. Tator CH, Fehlings MG, Thorpe K, et al. Current use and timing of spinal surgery for management of acute spinal surgery for management of acute spinal cord injury in North America: results of a retrospective multicenter study. J Neurosurg 1999;91(1 Suppl):12–8.
11. Wilson JR, Grossman RG, Frankowski RF, et al. A clinical prediction model for long-term functional outcome after traumatic spinal cord injury based on acute clinical and imaging factors. J Neurotrauma 2012;29(13):2263–71.
12. Mothe AJ, Tassew NG, Shabanzadeh AP, et al. RGMa inhibition with human monoclonal antibodies promotes regeneration, plasticity and repair, and attenuates neuropathic pain after spinal cord injury. Sci Rep 2017;7(1):10529.
13. Mothe AJ, Coelho M, Huang L, et al. Delayed administration of the human anti-RGMa monoclonal antibody elezanumab promotes functional recovery including spontaneous voiding after spinal cord injury in rats. Neurobiol Dis 2020;143:104995.
14. Koyanagi I, Tator CH, Lea PJ. Three-dimensional analysis of the vascular system in the rat spinal cord with scanning electron microscopy of vascular corrosion casts. Part 2: acute spinal cord injury. Neurosurgery 1993;33(2):285–91 [discussion: 292].
15. Weiss S, Dunne C, Hewson J, et al. Multipotent CNS stem cells are present in the adult mammalian spinal cord and ventricular neuroaxis. J Neurosci 1996; 16(23):7599–609.

16. Kojima A, Tator CH. Epidermal growth factor and fibroblast growth factor 2 cause proliferation of ependymal precursor cells in the adult rat spinal cord in vivo. J Neuropathol Exp Neurol 2000;59(8): 687–97.

17. Kojima A, Tator CH. Intrathecal administration of epidermal growth factor and fibroblast growth factor 2 promotes ependymal proliferation and functional recovery after spinal cord injury in adult rats. J Neurotrauma 2002;19(2):223–38.

18. Hachem LD, Mothe AJ, Tator CH. Unlocking the paradoxical endogenous stem cell response after spinal cord injury. Stem Cells 2020;38(2): 187–94.

19. Tator CH. Catastrophic injuries in sports and recreation, causes and prevention: a Canadian study. Toronto: University of Toronto Press; 2008. p. 761.

20. Chen Y, Tang Y, Allen V, et al. Fall-induced spinal cord injury: external causes and implications for prevention. J Spinal Cord Med 2016;39(1):24–31.

21. Selvarajah S, Hammond ER, Haider AH, et al. The burden of acute traumatic spinal cord injury among adults in the united states: an update. J Neurotrauma 2014;31(3):228–38.

Section I: Basics of SCI

Pathophysiology of Spinal Cord Injury

Laureen D. Hachem, MD[a,b], Michael G. Fehlings, MD, PhD[a,b],*

KEYWORDS

- Spinal cord injury • Pathogenesis • Secondary injury • Plasticity • Neural circuits

KEY POINTS

- The pathogenesis of spinal cord injury (SCI) is composed of a primary mechanical insult followed by a secondary cascade of cellular and molecular events, which further propagate tissue damage.
- The secondary chemical injury of SCI can be divided into acute, subacute, and chronic phases.
- Damage to host neurons leads to the loss of important neural relay circuits controlling respiration, locomotion, bladder function, and autonomic regulation.
- After SCI, endogenous repair mechanisms lead to the generation of new neural connections that underlie both adaptive and maladaptive plasticity.
- Understanding alterations in global neural networks, injury-dependent mediators of cell fate, and pathophysiological variation across heterogeneous injury patterns are areas of clinical priority in SCI.

INTRODUCTION

Spinal cord injury (SCI) triggers a complex cascade of molecular and chemical events that leads to progressive cell loss and tissue damage.[1,2] Nearly a century of fundamental basic science research has uncovered important mechanisms underlying the pathophysiology of SCI and informed the development of promising experimental treatment strategies. However, effective clinical translation of these therapies has required further study into the spatial and temporal integration of injury-induced signaling cascades, the heterogeneity in pathogenesis across injury patterns along with global neural network-level changes that occur after SCI. The advent of novel genetic techniques, advanced imaging modalities, and circuit interrogation strategies in recent years has facilitated the discovery of complex cellular interactions and network changes after SCI that has transformed our understanding of the dynamic injury environment.

Herein, the authors review the temporal profile of SCI pathogenesis, focusing on key molecular and cellular mediators of the secondary injury. They highlight cutting edge insights on the alterations in neural circuits that occur after SCI and describe how these changes largely define the chronic injury environment. They bridge these important basic science concepts with clinical implications for informing novel experimental therapies. Lastly, emerging concepts in the study of SCI pathogenesis that are transforming fundamental research into innovative clinical treatment paradigms are outlined.

PHASES OF INJURY

The initial primary mechanical injury that leads to SCI can result from a variety of mechanisms including compression, contusion, transection, and shearing forces.[3] Historically the typical phenotype of SCI was a high energy mechanism in young patients, resulting in severe cord damage and a complete neurologic injury. However, with a rapidly aging population, an increasing proportion of SCIs is seen in older patients due to minor traumas on a background of chronic compression

a Division of Neurosurgery, Department of Surgery, University of Toronto, 149 College Street, Toronto, Ontario M5T 1P5, Canada; b Division of Neurosurgery, Toronto Western Hospital, University Health Network, 399 Bathurst Street, Suite 4W-449, Toronto, Ontario M5T 2S8, Canada
* Corresponding author. 399 Bathurst Street, Suite 4W-449, Toronto, Ontario M5T 2S8, Canada.
E-mail address: Michael.Fehlings@uhn.ca

Neurosurg Clin N Am 32 (2021) 305–313
https://doi.org/10.1016/j.nec.2021.03.002
1042-3680/21/© 2021 Elsevier Inc. All rights reserved.

from degenerative cervical myelopathy, resulting in incomplete injuries.[4] Nevertheless, the primary mechanical insult that leads to cord compression triggers a complex cascade of molecular and cellular events, termed the secondary injury, that further propagates tissue damage. In order to mitigate these effects, current clinical practice guidelines recommend early decompressive surgery in the setting of ongoing compression after SCI.[5]

The secondary injury of SCI is divided into acute, subacute, and chronic stages (**Table 1**).[6] The acute injury environment, comprising the first 48 hours after SCI, is characterized by sudden alterations in ion homeostasis, release of reactive oxygen species, and excess excitatory neurotransmitters that overwhelm endogenous cellular repair systems leading to extensive neuronal and glial cell death. A large inflammatory response also ensues marked by increased blood-spinal cord barrier permeability and the infiltration of circulating leukocytes. The subacute period, lasting up to 2 weeks after SCI, is characterized by maturation of the injury site with development of a glial scar around the lesion epicenter and release of growth inhibitory molecules—critical events that influence the capacity for endogenous regeneration. The chronic stage of SCI is largely defined by remodeling of sparred circuits and regeneration of new neural networks that contribute to both adaptive and maladaptive plasticity.

MOLECULAR AND CHEMICAL MEDIATORS OF SPINAL CORD INJURY PATHOGENESIS
Ischemia and Vascular Mediators

A lack of adequate blood flow to the spinal cord due to impaired vascular regulation and systemic hypotension after SCI is a major contributor to injury. Within seconds of cord hypoperfusion, cellular adenosine triphosphate (ATP) stores become depleted leading to mitochondrial dysfunction and cell death. Furthermore, disruption of the blood-spinal cord barrier leads to vasogenic edema and impaired blood flow. Direct

compression along with central hemorrhage and local vasospasm further propagates the cascade of ischemic events.[7] In order to mitigate these effects, current guidelines recommend maintaining a mean arterial pressure greater than 85 mm Hg in the first week after SCI.[8] The importance of maintaining adequate spinal cord perfusion is further borne out by clinical studies demonstrating that a spinal cord perfusion pressure (SCPP) greater than 50 mm Hg is a predictor of improved neurologic recovery after SCI.[9] SCPP may therefore be a useful parameter to guide the management of patients with SCI in clinical practice.

Excitotoxicity and Ion Imbalance

Ion imbalance is a key hallmark of the secondary injury of SCI. Direct mechanical injury to host cells triggers the release of high concentrations of excitatory neurotransmitters that in turn induce large influxes in intracellular calcium in neuronal and glial cells, activating downstream apoptotic pathways.[10,11] Intracellular sodium concentrations also increase due to excess sodium influx via voltage-gated Na channels and a lack of efficient efflux from dysfunctional Na-K ATPases. This results in progressive acidosis and cytotoxic cellular edema.

Much of the research on ion homeostasis and excitatory neurotransmitter alterations after SCI has focused on the acute injury period. However, the initial injury leads to long-lasting changes in the composition of ion channels and neurotransmitter receptors that impairs neuronal signaling and plasticity in the chronic phase.[12,13]

Oxidative Stress

The resultant ischemic damage and cellular dysregulation after SCI leads to the formation of free radicals such as reactive oxygen and reactive nitrogen species, which overwhelm normal cellular antioxidant systems.[14] Free radicals exert detrimental effects on mitochondrial function with alterations in mitochondrial bioenergetics occurring within hours of injury.[15] Mitochondrial dysfunction leads to the production of toxic mediators and

Table 1
Primary and secondary injury mechanisms after traumatic SCI

Primary Injury	Secondary Injury		
	Acute	Subacute	Chronic
• Compression • Contusion • Transection • Shear	• Hypotension & Ischemia • Excitotoxicity & Ion imbalance • Oxidative stress • Inflammatory response • Edema	• Cellular apoptosis • Neurite growth inhibitory factors • Glial scar formation	• Altered neural circuitry • Syrinx formation

impairs the formation of ATP, which further propagates the initial insult. Targeting mitochondrial dysfunction has arisen as a promising treatment strategy in preclinical models of SCI.[16]

Inflammatory Response

Acute SCI leads to the production of cytokines and the infiltration of leukocytes into the injury site. A temporal pattern of immune cell recruitment is seen after SCI, with neutrophils infiltrating within the first few hours after injury, followed by microglia and peripheral monocyte-derived macrophages that persist at the site of injury for weeks.[17,18] The ensuing inflammatory cascade plays a dual role in tissue regeneration. Activated microglia secrete proinflammatory cytokines and cytotoxic factors that propagate cell death. Moreover, leukocyte infiltration leads to the production of matrix metalloproteinases, which degrade extracellular matrix components causing tissue injury, blood-spinal cord barrier disruption and edema.[19] Activated microglia induce the activity of a subtype of neurotoxic reactive astrocytes after SCI, which contribute to neuronal and glial cell death.[20] However, microglia are also necessary for the beneficial properties of the glial scar. Elimination of microglia in SCI animal models leads to aberrant scar formation, increased infiltration of peripheral myeloid cells, and increased tissue loss.[21]

Growth Inhibitory Factors

SCI causes upregulation of many inhibitory molecules that limit axonal growth and synaptic plasticity. Nogo-A, a glycosylated transmembrane protein, is the most widely studied of these molecules and exerts inhibitory effects on neurons via Nogo-66 and NiG domains. Anti-Nogo antibodies have demonstrated efficacy in improving locomotor recovery after SCI, and this strategy is currently under clinical investigation in SCI patients.[22,23] Targeting the downstream molecular pathways involved in growth inhibitory factor signaling has offered an alternative strategy to enhance regeneration after SCI. The intracellular GTPase RhoA and its downstream effector Rho-associated kinase are common targets of many myelin inhibitory proteins. Activation of the RhoA pathways inhibits actin cytoskeleton formation and limits axonal growth. Although Rho inhibitors have shown promise in preclinical SCI models, a recent clinical trial of a Rho inhibitor failed to show efficacy on interim analysis, thus leading to study termination.

Reactive Gliosis and Scar Formation

Acute SCI is associated with the activation of reactive astrocytes that form a large component of the glial scar surrounding the injury site. Although traditionally viewed as negative players in the pathogenesis of SCI, there is increasing evidence to suggest an important role of these cells in regeneration and recovery.[24] Indeed, blocking astrocytic scar formation reduces axon regrowth after SCI due to a reduction in axon growth–supporting molecules.[25] Furthermore, emerging evidence suggests that astrocytes may play a role in neurogenesis, whereby injury-related cues induce parenchymal astrocytes to generate new neurons.[26,27]

Despite the positive effects of the glial scar, several detrimental scar components serve as important targets for therapeutic design. The most widely studied of these molecules are chondroitin sulfate proteoglycans (CSPGs), which are secreted by reactive glia and inhibit axonal growth and plasticity. Chondroitinase is an enzyme that degrades the inhibitory CSPGs within the glial scar and has demonstrated promising results in large animal preclinical models of SCI.[28] Combinatorial approaches of chondroitinase with transplanted neural stem cells along with novel delivery platforms such as viral vector transgene delivery have emerged as strategies to target the negative effects of the glial scar and enhance regeneration after SCI.[29,30]

ALTERATIONS IN NEURAL CIRCUITRY

The biochemical and molecular cascade that comprises the acute and subacute stages of SCI leads to widespread neuronal and glial cell death, resulting in the disruption of neural circuits that control vital functions such as locomotion, respiration, and bladder regulation. The chronic phase of injury is consequently defined by a period of reorganization of sparred circuits and the development of new neural connections. Although this endogenous plasticity may serve as a substrate for spontaneous recovery, it also underlies many processes of aberrant rewiring of circuits (**Table 2**).

Autonomic Dysfunction

SCIs that occur above the T6 level disrupt descending control of thoracolumbar sympathetic preganglionic neurons (SPNs), resulting in autonomic dysreflexia. Several cellular mechanisms contribute to the development of this phenomenon. Initially, loss of supraspinal regulation of SPNs reduces sympathetic outflow. However, in the chronic stages of injury reorganization of neural circuitry results in hyperexcitability of SPNs and an exaggerated sympathetic reflex to peripheral stimuli. Excess sprouting of nociceptive C-fibers

Table 2
Alterations in neural circuitry following spinal cord injury

System	Pathophysiology
Autonomic regulation	• SCI above T6 disrupts descending control of SPNs • Initial loss of supraspinal regulation of SPNs reduces sympathetic outflow • Reorganization of neural circuitry results in hyperexcitability of SPNs • Excess sprouting of nociceptive C-fibers into the dorsal horn below the level of injury contributes to SPN hyperexcitability • Axonal sprouting in ascending propriospinal tracts carrying signals from the lumbosacral dorsal gray commissure promotes autonomic dysreflexia induced by bladder or colon distension
Respiratory control	• High cervical SCI causes axonal degeneration in phrenic nerve fibers controlling diaphragm function • Loss of supraspinal input to respiratory motor neurons controlling intercostal and abdominal muscles important for respiration • Spontaneous spinally derived phrenic motor rhythms are generated after SCI
Locomotor networks	• Alterations in CPG and reflex pathways occur below the level of injury • Decreased functional connectivity occurs between primary motor and sensory regions in the brain after SCI
Bladder regulation	• Recruitment of unmyelinated C fibers results in shorter latency period and neurogenic detrusor overactivity • Detrusor sphincter dyssynergia occurs, which leads to bladder outlet obstruction and bladder hypertrophy

Abbreviations: CPG, central pattern generator; SPN, sympathetic preganglionic neurons.

into the dorsal horn below the level of injury contributes to the hyperexcitability of SPNs via propriospinal relay neurons. Axonal sprouting is also seen in ascending propriospinal tracts carrying signals from the lumbosacral dorsal gray commissure, which likely underlies the dysreflexia seen with stimuli of bladder or colon distension.[31] Peripheral changes in catecholamine sensitivity following SCI further augment the aberrant circulatory response in autonomic dysreflexia.

Respiratory Circuitry

High cervical SCI leads to impairments in respiration due to axonal degeneration of phrenic nerve fibers controlling diaphragm function and the loss of supraspinal input to respiratory motor neurons controlling intercostal and abdominal muscles. Study into the respiratory circuit changes that occur after SCI has uncovered the possibility of spontaneous spinally derived phrenic motor rhythms. Indeed, phasic bursts occur in the phrenic motor neuron ipsilateral and caudal to C2 spinal injuries in rodents, and this pattern of firing is distinct from the preserved contralateral nerve, suggesting an inherent spinal rhythm that is uncovered in the

setting of injury.[32,33] Modulation of respiratory spinal rhythms may serve as a mechanism to enhance respiratory function after high cervical SCIs. Recently, stimulation of midcervical excitatory interneurons has been shown to maintain breathing in animal models of SCI.[34]

Locomotor Networks

Increasing evidence suggests a modular organization of locomotor circuits,[35] with both rhythm- and pattern-generating networks.[36,37] Studies in animal models of SCI have demonstrated a distinct temporal pattern of alterations in specific gait parameters after SCI with evidence of independent regulation of flexor and extensor components of spinal CPG control.[38] Understanding the complex regulation of spinal locomotor systems in both healthy and disease states has offered important targets for therapeutic design. Recent studies have uncovered a somatosensory cortical control of lumbar-activating rhythm-generating circuits by way of cervical excitatory interneurons in rodents, which may provide a target to modulate locomotion after injury.[39] Strategies to modulate locomotor networks after SCI by way of electrical stimulation,[40] brain controlled neuro-modulatory approaches,[41] and combinatorial pharmacological-stimulation paradigms hold promise for clinical translation.[42]

Bladder Regulation

Alteration in the micturition reflex forms the neural basis of bladder dysfunction after SCI. Under normal conditions, myelinated A delta fibers carry afferent information detecting bladder distension to the dorsal root ganglia.[43] Reorganization of synaptic connections following injury results in the recruitment of unmyelinated C fibers to relay reflex information, resulting in shorter latency periods and neurogenic detrusor overactivity. This is often coupled with detrusor sphincter dyssynergia, which leads to bladder outlet obstruction and subsequent bladder hypertrophy.[44]

Specific molecular targets have been identified in the pathogenesis of bladder dysfunction after SCI. Increased expression of the purinergic P2X3 receptor is seen in neurogenic bladders after SCI and P2X3 antagonists improve bladder function in animal models.[45] Furthermore, dysregulated proNGF/p75 signaling contributes to bladder dysfunction after SCI, with pharmacologic blockade of this pathway improving voiding reflexes.[46] Anti-RGMa antibody[47] and anti-Nogo[48] antibody have both shown positive results in reducing bladder dysfunction after SCI; however, the exact molecular mechanisms underlying these effects require further study. Novel electrical and magnetic stimulation neuromodulatory strategies are currently being investigated as additional strategies targeting bladder dysfunction after SCI.[49,50]

EMERGING CONCEPTS IN THE STUDY OF SPINAL CORD INJURY PATHOGENESIS
Bridging Injury Heterogeneity and Pathophysiology

Few studies on the pathophysiological mechanisms of SCI have considered the impact of injury severity, level, or mechanism on the underlying neurobiology. However, the heterogeneity seen across patients in injury phenotypes and clinical trajectories suggests that there are likely important differences at a molecular and cellular level.

Recent studies in rodent models of SCI have revealed level-dependent differences in the immune response between cervical and thoracic injuries. Specifically, cervical SCI is associated with reduced expression of proinflammatory and antiinflammatory proteins compared with thoracic injuries; this may in part be due to the sympathetic dysregulation seen with higher level SCIs.[51] Furthermore, the severity of injury leads to differences in sparred neural networks with complete transections producing more pronounced loss of supraspinal input, whereas mild injuries may lead to local deafferentation with relative preservation of supraspinal signals.[52] The resultant environment may impart differences in endogenous plasticity and repair responses.

The importance of understanding disease heterogeneity at a pathophysiological level is best demonstrated in the case of central cord injury. Although it was once thought that the disproportionate preservation of lower extremity compared with upper extremity function in this condition was due to a somatotopic organization of the corticospinal tract, increasing lines of evidence have challenged this concept.[53,54] Indeed, a somatotopic organization has not been found in humans, and instead, the resulting clinical picture is likely due to the preservation of extrapyramidal tracts that contribute to lower extremity function.[55]

Injury-Dependent Mediators of Cell Fate

Stem cell–based therapies have become an important strategy to promote the regeneration of damaged cells. Recent studies have begun to uncover critical injury–induced cues that direct the differentiation of both endogenous and transplanted stem cells to specific lineages. SCI activates Notch signaling in neural stem cells and promotes a differentiation switch to astrocytes. Strategies to block Notch signaling have subsequently been shown to enhance neuronal differentiation of transplanted stem cells and promote functional recovery.[56] Moreover, ErbB tyrosine kinase receptor signaling has been found to control oligodendrocyte progenitor cell transformation and spontaneous remyelination after SCI.[57] Recently, a latent lineage potential in endogenous spinal cord neural stem cells has been discovered that is uncovered only after injury and promotes differentiation toward an oligodendroglial fate.[58] Collectively, this work provides important targets to direct the differentiation of stem cells toward neuronal or oligodendroglial phenotypes in order to enhance the effectiveness of cellular therapies.

Beyond the Spinal Cord: Global Network Plasticity

Although discussions on the pathogenesis of SCI have historically focused on alterations within the spinal cord, there is robust evidence demonstrating important cortical changes that occur after SCI. These alterations in brain neural networks may have a profound impact on the course of plasticity and serve as potential biomarkers for treatment response.

Table 3
Therapeutic strategies targeting secondary injury mediators of spinal cord injury

Strategy	Mechanism	Stage of Study
Minocycline	• Mitochondrial stabilization and reduction in apoptotic pathway activation • Downregulation of TNFa, IL-1β, NOS	Clinical Trial (phase III)
Riluzole	• Inactivation of voltage-gated sodium channels • Increased reuptake of extracellular glutamate • Reduction in intracellular sodium and calcium along with extracellular glutamate	Clinical Trial (phase II/III)
Granulocyte colony-stimulating factor	• Suppression of proinflammatory cytokines, MMPs, and apoptotic pathways • Reduction in neutrophil infiltration • Recruitment and integration of progenitor cells at the injury site	Clinical Trial (phase I/II)
Anti-Nogo A antibody	• Inhibition of Nogo-A signaling by way of the Rho-ROCK pathway	Clinical Trial (phase II)
Stem cell transplantation	• Various cell sources under clinical trial including OPCs, Schwann cells, umbilical cord–derived stem cells, BMSCs • Replacement of lost neurons and oligodendrocytes, remyelination, secretion of beneficial trophic factors	Clinical Trial (various phases)
Hypothermia	• Reduction in free radicals and excitotoxic neurotransmitter release • Preservation of BSCB integrity, reduction in host inflammatory response • Induction of cold-induced proteins with neuroprotective properties	Clinical Trial
Chondroitinase	• Degradation of inhibitory CSPGs within the glial scar promoting axonal sprouting	Preclinical
Anti-RGMa antibody	• Blockade of inhibitory RGMa signaling via the Neogenin receptor • Enhances neuronal survival, plasticity, and CST axonal growth	Preclinical

Abbreviations: BMSC, bone marrow stromal cell; BSCB, blood-spinal cord barrier; CST, corticospinal tract; IL-1β, interleukin-1 beta; RGMa, repulsive guidance molecule a; TNFa, tumor necrosis factor alpha.

It has long been known that SCI induces reorganization of the motor and sensory cortex; however, advances in functional MRI techniques have added a deeper understanding to the network-level changes that occur after SCI. Both animal and human studies have reported decreased functional connections between primary motor and sensory regions in the brain after SCI. In contrast, increased connections form between the primary sensory cortex and caudoputamen/anterior cingulate pain–associated regions after SCI, suggesting a possible neural correlate for neuropathic pain responses.[59,60] Moreover, progressive atrophy and microstructural changes across motor and sensory systems seem to be correlated with clinical outcomes, which raises

the possibility of using these parameters as clinical biomarkers.[61,62]

SUMMARY

The complex cascade of molecular and chemical events that ensue following SCI create a hostile environment within the cord that induces widespread cell death and restricts tissue regeneration. Various components of this cascade have been the target of promising therapeutic strategies (**Table 3**) in preclinical models of SCI. With technological advances across the spectrum of genetic and molecular techniques and a growing toolbox to interrogate cortical and spinal circuits, the coming years will witness an acceleration in our understanding of fundamental injury processes in order to effectively translate experimental therapies to patients.

CLINICS CARE POINTS

- Maintaining adequate blood flow to the spinal cord along with early surgical decompression is of utmost importance in mitigating the acute effects of SCI.

- Neuroprotective and neuroregenerative therapies targeting the secondary injury cascade of SCI are on the horizon for clinical translation.

- Understanding the alterations in neural circuitry that occur after SCI offers insight into targeted therapies to rewire damaged neural networks and mitigate aberrant plasticity.

- Novel rehabilitation and electrical stimulation strategies offer promise in restoring damaged neural circuitry after SCI.

REFERENCES

1. Allen AR. Surgery for experimental lesions of spinal cord equivalent to crush injury of fracture dislocation of spinal column: a preliminary report. JAMA 1911; 57:878–80.
2. Tator CH, Fehlings MG. Review of the secondary injury theory of acute spinal cord trauma with emphasis on vascular mechanisms. J Neurosurg 1991;75(1):15–26.
3. Alizadeh A, Dyck SM, Karimi-Abdolrezaee S. Traumatic spinal cord injury: an overview of pathophysiology, models and acute injury mechanisms. Front Neurol 2019;10:282.
4. Wilson JR, Cronin S, Fehlings MG, et al. Epidemiology and impact of spinal cord injury in the elderly: results of a fifteen-year population-based cohort study. J Neurotrauma 2020;37(15):1740–51.
5. Fehlings MG, Vaccaro A, Wilson JR, et al. Early versus delayed decompression for traumatic cervical spinal cord injury: results of the Surgical Timing in Acute Spinal Cord Injury Study (STASCIS). PLoS One 2012;7(2):e32037.
6. Hachem LD, Ahuja CS, Fehlings MG. Assessment and management of acute spinal cord injury: from point of injury to rehabilitation. J Spinal Cord Med 2017;40(6):665–75.
7. Mautes AE, Weinzierl MR, Donovan F, et al. Vascular events after spinal cord injury: contribution to secondary pathogenesis. Phys Ther 2000;80(7):673–87.

8. Hawryluk G, Whetstone W, Saigal R, et al. Mean arterial blood pressure correlates with neurological recovery after human spinal cord injury: analysis of high frequency physiologic data. J Neurotrauma 2015;32(24):1958–67.
9. Squair JW, Bélanger LM, Tsang A, et al. Spinal cord perfusion pressure predicts neurologic recovery in acute spinal cord injury. Neurology 2017;89(16): 1660–7.
10. Xu GY, Hughes MG, Ye Z, et al. Concentrations of glutamate released following spinal cord injury kill oligodendrocytes in the spinal cord. Exp Neurol 2004;187(2):329–36.
11. Xu GY, Liu S, Hughes MG, et al. Glutamate-induced losses of oligodendrocytes and neurons and activation of caspase-3 in the rat spinal cord. Neuroscience 2008;153(4):1034–47.
12. Garcia VB, Abbinanti MD, Harris-Warrick RM, et al. Effects of chronic spinal cord injury on relationships among ion channel and receptor mrnas in mouse lumbar spinal cord. Neuroscience 2018;393:42–60.
13. Grossman SD, Wolfe BB, Yasuda RP, et al. Changes in NMDA receptor subunit expression in response to contusive spinal cord injury. J Neurochem 2000; 75(1):174–84.
14. Visavadiya NP, Patel SP, VanRooyen JL, et al. Cellular and subcellular oxidative stress parameters following severe spinal cord injury. Redox Biol 2016; 8:59–67.
15. Sullivan PG, Krishnamurthy S, Patel SP, et al. Temporal characterization of mitochondrial bioenergetics after spinal cord injury. J Neurotrauma 2007;24(6):991–9.
16. Rabchevsky AG, Michael FM, Patel SP. Mitochondria focused neurotherapeutics for spinal cord injury. Exp Neurol 2020;330:113332.
17. Greenhalgh AD, David S. Differences in the phagocytic response of microglia and peripheral macrophages after spinal cord injury and its effects on cell death. J Neurosci 2014;34(18):6316–22.
18. Okada S. The pathophysiological role of acute inflammation after spinal cord injury. Inflamm Regen 2016;36:20.
19. Noble LJ, Donovan F, Igarashi T, et al. Matrix metalloproteinases limit functional recovery after spinal cord injury by modulation of early vascular events. J Neurosci 2002;22(17):7526–35.
20. Liddelow SA, Guttenplan KA, Clarke LE, et al. Neurotoxic reactive astrocytes are induced by activated microglia. Nature 2017;541(7638):481–7.
21. Bellver-Landete V, Bretheau F, Mailhot B, et al. Microglia are an essential component of the neuroprotective scar that forms after spinal cord injury. Nat Commun 2019;10(1):518.
22. Chen K, Marsh BC, Cowan M, et al. Sequential therapy of anti-Nogo-A antibody treatment and treadmill training leads to cumulative improvements after spinal cord injury in rats. Exp Neurol 2017;292:135–44.

23. Kucher K, Johns D, Maier D, et al. First-in-man intrathecal application of neurite growth-promoting anti-nogo-a antibodies in acute spinal cord injury. Neurorehabil Neural Repair 2018;32(6–7):578–89.

24. Bradbury EJ, Burnside ER. Moving beyond the glial scar for spinal cord repair. Nat Commun 2019;10(1): 3879.

25. Anderson MA, Burda JE, Ren Y, et al. Astrocyte scar formation aids central nervous system axon regeneration. Nature 2016;532(7598):195–200.

26. Magnusson JP, Zamboni M, Santopolo G, et al. Activation of a neural stem cell transcriptional program in parenchymal astrocytes. Elife 2020;9:e59733.

27. Zamboni M, Llorens-Bobadilla E, Magnusson JP, et al. A widespread neurogenic potential of neocortical astrocytes is induced by injury. Cell Stem Cell 2020; 27(4):605–17.

28. Rosenzweig ES, Salegio EA, Liang JJ, et al. Chondroitinase improves anatomical and functional outcomes after primate spinal cord injury. Nat Neurosci 2019;22(8):1269–75.

29. Burnside ER, De Winter F, Didangelos A, et al. Immune-evasive gene switch enables regulated delivery of chondroitinase after spinal cord injury. Brain 2018;141(8):2362–81.

30. Suzuki H, Ahuja CS, Salewski RP, et al. Neural stem cell mediated recovery is enhanced by Chondroitinase ABC pretreatment in chronic cervical spinal cord injury. PLoS One 2017;12(8):e0182339.

31. Eldahan KC, Rabchevsky AG. Autonomic dysreflexia after spinal cord injury: Systemic pathophysiology and methods of management. Auton Neurosci 2018;209:59–70.

32. Sunshine MD, Sutor TW, Fox EJ, et al. Targeted activation of spinal respiratory neural circuits. Exp Neurol 2020;328:113256.

33. Ghali MG, Marchenko V. Patterns of phrenic nerve discharge after complete high cervical spinal cord injury in the decerebrate rat. J Neurotrauma 2016; 33(12):1115–27.

34. Satkunendrarajah K, Karadimas SK, Laliberte AM, et al. Cervical excitatory neurons sustain breathing after spinal cord injury. Nature 2018;562(7727): 419–22.

35. Bellardita C, Kiehn O. Phenotypic characterization of speed-associated gait changes in mice reveals modular organization of locomotor networks. Curr Biol 2015;25(11):1426–36.

36. Pocratsky AM, Burke DA, Morehouse JR, et al. Reversible silencing of lumbar spinal interneurons unmasks a task-specific network for securing hindlimb alternation. Nat Commun 2017;8(1):1963.

37. Kiehn O. Decoding the organization of spinal circuits that control locomotion. Nat Rev Neurosci 2016; 17(4):224–38.

38. Martinez M, Delivet-Mongrain H, Leblond H, et al. Incomplete spinal cord injury promotes durable functional changes within the spinal locomotor circuitry. J Neurophysiol 2012;108(1):124–34.

39. Karadimas SK, Satkunendrarajah K, Laliberte AM, et al. Sensory cortical control of movement. Nat Neurosci 2020;23(1):75–84.

40. Marquez-Chin C, Popovic MR. Functional electrical stimulation therapy for restoration of motor function after spinal cord injury and stroke: a review. Biomed Eng Online 2020;19(1):34.

41. Bonizzato M, Pidpruzhnykova G, DiGiovanna J, et al. Brain-controlled modulation of spinal circuits improves recovery from spinal cord injury. Nat Commun 2018;9(1):3015.

42. Taccola G, Salazar BH, Apicella R, et al. Selective Antagonism of A1 adenosinergic receptors strengthens the neuromodulation of the sensorimotor network during epidural spinal stimulation. Front Syst Neurosci 2020;14:44.

43. Hamid R, Averbeck MA, Chiang H, et al. Epidemiology and pathophysiology of neurogenic bladder after spinal cord injury. World J Urol 2018;36(10): 1517–27.

44. de Groat WC, Yoshimura N. Mechanisms underlying the recovery of lower urinary tract function following spinal cord injury. Prog Brain Res 2006;152:59–84.

45. Andersson KE. Potential future pharmacological treatment of bladder dysfunction. Basic Clin Pharmacol Toxicol 2016;119(Suppl 3):75–85.

46. Ryu JC, Tooke K, Malley SE, et al. Role of proNGF/p75 signaling in bladder dysfunction after spinal cord injury. J Clin Invest 2018;128(5):1772–86.

47. Mothe AJ, Coelho M, Huang L, et al. Delayed administration of the human anti-RGMa monoclonal antibody elezanumab promotes functional recovery including spontaneous voiding after spinal cord injury in rats. Neurobiol Dis 2020;143:104995.

48. Schneider MP, Sartori AM, Ineichen BV, et al. Anti-Nogo-A antibodies as a potential causal therapy for lower urinary tract dysfunction after spinal cord injury. J Neurosci 2019;39(21):4066–76.

49. Niu T, Bennett CJ, Keller TL, et al. A proof-of-concept study of transcutaneous magnetic spinal cord stimulation for neurogenic bladder. Sci Rep 2018;8(1):12549.

50. Kreydin E, Zhong H, Latack K, et al. Transcutaneous Electrical Spinal Cord Neuromodulator (TESCoN) improves symptoms of overactive bladder. Front Syst Neurosci 2020;14:1.

51. Hong J, Chang A, Zavvarian MM, et al. Level-specific differences in systemic expression of pro- and anti-inflammatory cytokines and chemokines after spinal cord injury. Int J Mol Sci 2018;19(8): 2167.

52. Hong J, Chang A, Liu Y, et al. Incomplete spinal cord injury reverses the level-dependence of spinal cord injury immune deficiency syndrome. Int J Mol Sci 2019;20(15):3762.

53. Lawrence DG, Kuypers HG. The functional organization of the motor system in the monkey. I. The effects of bilateral pyramidal lesions. Brain 1968; 91(1):1–14.

54. Quencer RM, Bunge RP, Egnor M, et al. Acute traumatic central cord syndrome: MRI-pathological correlations. Neuroradiology 1992;34(2):85–94.

55. Levi AD, Tator CH, Bunge RP. Clinical syndromes associated with disproportionate weakness of the upper versus the lower extremities after cervical spinal cord injury. Neurosurgery 1996;38(1):179–83 [discussion 83-5].

56. Khazaei M, Ahuja CS, Nakashima H, et al. GDNF rescues the fate of neural progenitor grafts by attenuating Notch signals in the injured spinal cord in rodents. Sci Transl Med 2020;12(525): eaau3538.

57. Bartus K, Burnside ER, Galino J, et al. ErbB receptor signaling directly controls oligodendrocyte progenitor cell transformation and spontaneous remyelination after spinal cord injury. Glia 2019;67(6): 1036–46.

58. Llorens-Bobadilla E, Chell JM, Le Merre P, et al. A latent lineage potential in resident neural stem cells enables spinal cord repair. Science 2020; 370(6512):eabb8795.

59. Matsubayashi K, Nagoshi N, Komaki Y, et al. Assessing cortical plasticity after spinal cord injury by using resting-state functional magnetic resonance imaging in awake adult mice. Sci Rep 2018;8(1): 14406.

60. Oni-Orisan A, Kaushal M, Li W, et al. Alterations in cortical sensorimotor connectivity following complete cervical spinal cord injury: a prospective resting-state fMRI Study. PLoS One 2016;11(3): e0150351.

61. Grabher P, Callaghan MF, Ashburner J, et al. Tracking sensory system atrophy and outcome prediction in spinal cord injury. Ann Neurol 2015;78(5): 751–61.

62. Chen Q, Zheng W, Chen X, et al. Brain gray matter atrophy after spinal cord injury: a voxel-based morphometry study. Front Hum Neurosci 2017; 11:211.

The Natural History of Spinal Cord Injury

Alexander F. Haddad, BS, John F. Burke, MD, PhD, Sanjay S. Dhall, MD*

KEYWORDS

- Natural history • Spinal cord injury • SCI

KEY POINTS

- The natural history of spinal cord injury remains elusive because of limitations in determine injury severity at the time of initial diagnosis, improving rehabilitation techniques, and devices that assist with community re-integration.
- Five percent to 20% of patients with a complete spinal cord injury will convert to an incomplete injury.
- However, meaningful functional recovery is very rare in patients with complete spinal cord injury compared with those with incomplete spinal cord injury.
- New technology and therapies are changing how we evaluate and treat patients with spinal cord injury.

INTRODUCTION

The complex function of the spinal cord, combined with its relatively delicate composition of long thin cellular processes and predisposition to damaging inflammatory responses, make it exceptionally susceptible to injury.[1] Spinal cord injury (SCI) negatively affects transmission of motor and sensory information through the level of the injury. An SCI can have a devastating impact on patient quality of life; afflicted patients experience a range of symptoms, including paralysis, respiratory and cardiovascular failure, decreased sexual function, and severe reflex spasms.[2,3] Initial attempts to study SCI were hampered by the lack of consistency in classification schemes and standardized outcomes across studies. This subsequently led to attempts to create unified grading schemes with which to describe SCI, culminating in 1992 with the American Spinal Injury Association (ASIA) SCI Impairment Scale (AIS) and its revisions.[4,5] The ASIA classification scheme has allowed for more precise clinical investigations into SCI including those pertaining to epidemiology and outcomes, as well as the natural history of SCI.

Despite the incredible morbidity associated with SCI, there remains a paucity of large-scale research endeavors in the field. Yet in the United States alone, 17,000 people are afflicted with SCI each year, a number that is likely under-reported.[3] For reference, other major neurosurgical diseases, such as glioblastoma (12,000/y), operative meningiomas (15,000/y), ruptured arteriovenous malformations (3000/y), and spinal cord tumors (2700/y) each afflict fewer patients. In addition to crippling physical limitations, SCI comes with a high economic burden associated with it. For example, in contrast with patients with glioblastoma, patients with an SCI have survival rates approaching those of the normal population, but with a lifetime of incredible disability. The high prevalence of patients with an SCI (estimated to be 240,000–347,000 in the United States) with estimated lifetime direct costs of $1.1 to $4.7 million dollars per patient contribute to a total economic strain

Department of Neurological Surgery, University of California, San Francisco, 505 Parnassus Avenue, M779, San Francisco, CA 94143, USA
* Corresponding author.
E-mail address: Sanjay.Dhall@ucsf.edu

Neurosurg Clin N Am 32 (2021) 315–321
https://doi.org/10.1016/j.nec.2021.03.003
1042-3680/21/© 2021 Elsevier Inc. All rights reserved.

of $267 to $1631 billion from this condition. The physical, emotional, and economic burdens associated with SCI highlight the importance of better understanding this disease.

In this article, we discuss the natural history of SCI, including historical thinking and newer developments in the field. We also discuss the paucity of SCI research, difficulties associated with current SCI research, and potential future directions of investigation.

THE NATURAL HISTORY OF SPINAL CORD INJURY

Historically, the natural history of SCI has been viewed with a pessimistic lens, given the lack of improvement seen in many patients after injury, despite treatment.[6] But SCI prognosis can also be quite variable owing to differences in the mechanism of injury, severity, and level of injury, all of which can impact subsequent AIS grade conversion rates. Additional confounding variables obscuring the natural history of SCI include heterogeneity in outcome measures used across studies and the timing of outcome measures, because most of the recovery in both complete and incomplete SCI occurs within the first 6 to 9 months after an injury.[7,8] As a result, the natural history of SCI remains an open question. However, it is often held that complete SCI, in which there is no motor or sensory function below the level of injury, represents an irrecoverable injury, whereas incomplete injuries harbor the possibility of recovery. Although this general concept may seem like an oversimplification, many spinal surgeons will use this "rule of thumb" to make operative decisions for SCI. Given this circumstance, here we discuss the natural history of both complete and incomplete injuries.

COMPLETE SPINAL CORD INJURIES

A significant determinant of prognosis after SCI is the initial AIS grade, with AIS A patients having much lower rates of improvement. Although a general lack of data exists surrounding the historical conversion rate from AIS A to less severe grades of injury, the literature reports approximately 5% to 20% of patients will improve at least 1 grade. However, meaningful functional recovery, such as the ability to walk, is exceedingly rare.[4,5,9] A number of retrospective studies have sought to further define the prognosis of patients with an AIS A injury. In a 1999 study from the US Model Spinal Cord Injury System, Marino and colleagues[10] reported a 13% conversion rate from AIS A in patients admitted within 1 week of injury.

However, only 2.3% of patients converted to AIS D, highlighting the limited degree of meaningful functional recovery. A subsequent review by Fawcett and colleagues[11] reported a 20% conversion rate in AIS A patients, with 10% converting to AIS B and 10% converting to AIS C. Interestingly, tetraplegic patients were almost twice as likely to have some recovery when compared with paraplegic patients, although the reasoning for this finding was unclear.[11] In a more recent meta-analysis of 11 randomized clinical trials and 9 observational studies, El Tecle and colleagues[5] reported the overall conversion rate to be 28% in AIS A patients. Patients undergoing early surgery (defined as surgery within 24 hours of injury) had a significantly higher rate of conversion (46% vs 25%), relative to those undergoing late surgery, possibly indicating a benefit to early surgery. This finding also corresponds with a study by Burke and colleagues,[12] demonstrating significantly higher rates of conversion in AIS A patients after ultra-early surgical decompression. Nevertheless, the conversion rates described by El Tecle and associates[5] in both early and late surgical candidates are higher than what has previously been described, perhaps reflecting benefit of modern rehabilitation methods.

When interpreting the results of studies reporting the natural history or impact of treatment on SCI, it is also critical to consider additional variables, such as the timing of the initial examination, the presence of distracting factors during the initial examination, and the timeframe of recovery. Indeed, the timing of the initial examination can have a significant impact on reported conversion rates, because many improvements in functional status happen early in the course of the injury.[13] This result is highlighted in 2 studies by Waters and colleagues,[14,15] where complete SCI was defined based on a neurologic examination 1 month after injury; much lower conversion rates (4%–10%) were observed than traditionally described, demonstrating the importance of timing on the initial examination and highlighting the amount of recovery that can happen in the first 30 days after an injury. A subsequent study including 571 patients with complete spinal cord injuries by Kirshblum and colleagues[16] investigated late conversion (between 1- and 5-years after an injury). They found that only 5.6% of AIS A patients had any improvement during that recovery timeframe. Of the 2% who converted to motor incomplete status, only 3 patients improved to AIS D (0.5%).[16]

Circumstances surrounding the initial evaluation of a patient can also impact the accuracy of an evaluation. Burns and colleagues[17] highlighted this phenomenon in their study of 103 patients with an SCI by showing that patients with distracting comorbidities impacting cognition or communication had higher rates of conversion (17.4% vs 6.7%) and recovery of motor function (13.0% vs 0%) at 1 year or later when compared with patients without factors impacting examination reliability. As a result, the reliability of the initial examination should also be considered when interpreting conversion rates.

Although conversion from AIS A to other AIS grades is an important metric demonstrating recovery, it is also vital to consider recovery on a more granular level indicated by specific myotomes and dermatomes. This strategy can allow for a more comprehensive understanding of the overall clinical trajectory and more accurate patient counseling. The second National Acute Spinal Cord Injury Study (NASCIS) comparing methylprednisolone and naloxone with placebo for the treatment of acute SCI reported detailed motor, pinprick, and light touch scores for patients, providing significant insight into limb-specific recovery.[18,19] Despite optimism over AIS grade conversion rates, these data highlight the much more sobering prognosis for meaningful functional recovery in AIS A patients. By definition, all AIS A patients start with a motor score of 0. On a scale of 0 to 70, NASCIS II placebo AIS A patients achieved total motor scores of 1.3 points at 6 weeks, 4.2 points at 6 months, and ultimately 4.6 points at 1 year of follow-up.[18,19] This improvement is not quite enough return of function to convert 1 muscle from paralysis to normal strength (5 points), but of course is even further diluted because the improvement is spread out over 7 to 14 muscle groups below the level of the injury. Sensation testing (scored 29–87) also demonstrated minimal change in AIS A patients, improving 2.2, 2.6, and 4.0 points in pinprick, and 4.7, 5.1, and 5.5 points in light touch at the same time intervals—also spread out over all of the dermatomes below the level of the injury. Although NASCIS II was performed in the late 1980s and early 1990s and might underestimate the amount of functional ability that can be recovered with modern rehabilitation techniques, it still provides valuable insight into the trajectory of patients with an SCI and acts a benchmark historical control (**Table 1**).

INCOMPLETE SPINAL CORD INJURIES

When compared with patients with a complete SCI, patients with an incomplete SCI (AIS B–D) have significantly better conversion rates and functional outcomes.[9,20] This finding may represent a difference in the underlying pathophysiology between incomplete and complete SCIs. More severely injured patients with complete SCI may have few to no intact axons after injury, limiting their ability to recover functionally and "trapping" them in a plateau of limited recovery potential (**Fig. 1**).[21,22]

In a systematic review and meta-analysis of 114 studies, Khorasanizadeh and colleagues[20] highlighted the differences in conversion rates between various ASIA/Frankel classifications, demonstrating significantly lower rates of conversion in AIS A patients (19%) relative to those with grades B (74%), C (87%), and D (47%) injuries. They postulate that the lower incidence of conversion in AIS D patients is due to a "ceiling" effect, limiting the amount of recovery for these patients with relatively less severe injuries.[20] These results are also seen in a study of 460 acute patients with an SCI by Curt and colleagues,[23] who demonstrated improved functional recovery over 12 months in patients with an incomplete SCI relative to patients with a complete SCI, as well as improved functional recovery in patients with lower AIS grades, relative to more severe injuries. Similarly, Waters and colleagues[24,25] have demonstrated a relationship between strength at 1 month after injury and the degree of recovery at 1 year after injury in both tetraplegic and paraplegic patients. This finding may indicate a subset of patients with initial complete SCI at the time of injury, but enough intact axons to allow them to at least partially climb the recovery curve at 1 month and beyond (see **Fig. 1**). Results of the second NASCIS also demonstrate higher functional recovery scores in patients with incomplete SCIs relative to patients with complete SCIs, further emphasizing the improved prognosis of this patient population (see **Table 1**).[18,19,26]

RECOVERY OF WALKING ABILITY AFTER SPINAL CORD INJURY

In addition to recovery of bowel and bladder function, patients with an SCI and treating physicians alike view the recovery of walking function as a significant goal. A study by Ditunno and colleagues involving both providers and patients demonstrated the high importance of walking ability to both groups, ranking it among the most desirable functions, along with bowel and bladder function.[9,27] Not surprisingly, questions regarding regaining the ability to walk frequently arise within the SCI patient population, highlighting the importance of research in this arena as well as provider knowledge regarding the natural history

Table 1
Summary of SCI natural history outcomes

Complete or Incomplete	Conversion Rate	NASCIS 1-Year Functional Improvement: Motor[a]	NASCIS 1-Year Functional Improvement: Pinprick[b]	NASCIS One Year Functional Improvement-Light Touch[b]
Complete	AIS A: 5%–20%	4.6	5.1	5.5
Incomplete	AIS B: 74% AIS C: 87% AIS D: 47%	31.3 12.9	15.8 9.2	10.8 3.0

[a] Motor scored from 0 to 70.
[b] Pinprick and light touch scored from 29 to 87.

surrounding the recovery of this key function. In this section, we briefly discuss patient and injury characteristics that predict ambulation, including initial neurologic examination, age, and injury etiology.

As pointed out elsewhere in this article, the initial neurologic examination and AIS grade are the strongest predictors of neurologic recovery, with motor incomplete injuries faring best.[20] However, although it has been used as an outcome in a number of clinical trials, there is a paucity of studies linking AIS grade improvement with the ability to walk, arguing the need for ambulation to be included as a distinct functional outcome. A 2009 study of 273 patients by Van Middendorp and colleagues[28] sought to further define the relationship between AIS and walking ability. They reported that AIS conversion in motor complete patients did not correlate with the ability to walk; less than 15% of those who improved in grade from AIS A regained the ability to walk.[16] Furthermore, the level of injury was not provided for these

patients; previous research has shown that AIS A patients who recover the ability to walk (frequently with the use of braces) are often those with injuries in the region of the conus.[29] Similar discordance between AIS conversion and walking ability was noted in other AIS grades as well.[9,28]

Additional variables impacting the recovery of the functional ability to walk can vary depending on AIS status of the patient. In patients with AIS B injuries, a number of studies have implicated the ability to sense pinprick sensation (as opposed to light touch alone) in the recovery of walking, perhaps indicating less damage in proximity to white matter tracts subserving ambulation.[9] In AIS C patients, age correlates inversely with the ability to regain walking function; patients more than 50 years of age have nearly one-half the chance of ambulating relative to patients less than 50 years of age. The underlying reason for this is unclear, but may be related to decreased functional reserve or neuronal plasticity.[9,30]

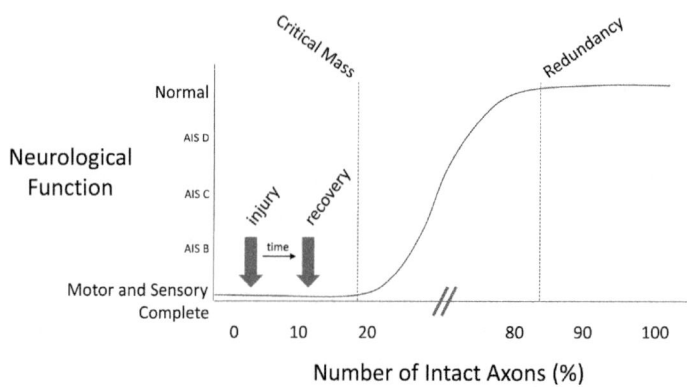

Fig. 1. Neurologic function as a derivative of the population of intact axons in the spinal cord. A critical mass of intact axons is required (estimated at 20% for illustrative purposes) before further increases in surviving axons can translate to neurologic improvement. Recovery of an additional 10% of the axon pool when only 10% are operational will not result in any detectable clinical improvement. This may explain why patients with severe SCI (motor and sensory complete) carry such a poor prognosis. At the other end of the spectrum, the graph also demonstrates the ceiling effect for improvement in AIS D patients: only 80% of axons may be required for normal or near-normal function, above which axonal recovery cannot be measured clinically.

NEUROMODULATION AFTER SPINAL CORD INJURY

Perhaps one of the most significant developments in the natural history of SCI has been the application of neuromodulation technology to those with chronic SCI injuries. In brief, this area of research has transformed how we think about the natural history of SCI. Patients with chronic SCI can show signs of functional improvement years after injury by means of epidural electrode implantation and stimulation below their injury site in the lumbo-sacral region.[31,32] Epidural stimulation has been shown to improve overground walking in patients who were previously paralyzed.[31,33,34]

The biological principle behind such neuromodulation is thought to be the central pattern generator.[35,36] This hypothetical circuit exists within the spinal cord and is capable of supporting ambulation in the absence of any information or neural signaling from higher level structures, hence facilitating our ability to walk without thinking. Practically, the central pattern generator in humans has been shown to be modulated by epidural stimulation and gait training,[37,38] which can be supplied in tandem to patients with complete SCI to activate central pattern generators, resulting in ambulation. This technology is currently in its infancy and is becoming increasingly more complex. Closed loop stimulation paradigms are being proposed to improve motor and ambulatory recovery.[39] An excellent summary can be found in the Iahn Cajigas and Aditya Vedantam's article, "Brain Computer Interface, Neuromodulation, and Neurorehabilitation Strategies for Spinal Cord Injury," in this issue.

FUTURE DIRECTIONS

There is an urgent need for bigger and better data detailing acute SCI treatments and outcomes on a national and even global scale. Multicenter databases can address some of these deficiencies by providing large, standardized datasets from heterogenous patient populations that can be interrogated to answer number of clinical questions. The International Spinal Cord Society and ASIA formed a global collaboration in 2002 to build a database using standard SCI variables known as the International SCI Data Set.[4] The National Institute of Neurologic Disorders and Stroke developed their own Common Data Elements project in 2006, which facilitates systematic data collection and analysis techniques on a number of neurologic disorders including SCI, and providing an excellent resource for researchers.[40] Building on this work, in 2013 the Department of Defense launched a multicenter, observational patient registry: Transforming Research and Clinical Knowledge in SCI (TRACK-SCI). TRACK-SCI uses SCI Common Data Elements to establish a dataset of granular patient data, including information on clinical and radiographic patient characteristics, blood biomarkers, and clinical interventions; it also includes information on a broad spectrum of neurologic, psychological, and functional outcomes.[2,41,42]

Well-organized and -established infrastructures such as TRACK-SCI will eventually allow for large-scale and rapid testing of new interventions for SCI such as neuromodulation and hypothermia. Standardized datasets will also facilitate more accurate investigation into the epidemiology and natural history of SCI, providing better targets and outcome measures for subsequent translational trials. Improved infrastructure surrounding local SCI research will also facilitate higher quality multicenter clinical trials. Although additional work is required to improve the culture and conditions surrounding SCI research, the future continues to hold great promise for our patients.

SUMMARY

The natural history of SCI is in a state of flux: the historical epidemiology of SCI is currently being reshaped by emerging treatments and technologies. Residual motor function after injury remains the best predictor for degree of recovery; the less severe the motor deficit, the greater the chance for meaningful improvement in both strength and sensation, occurring over a period of 6 to 9 months. AIS grade conversion does not equate to the ability to ambulate. An important part of the future for SCI research is big data in the form of national and international registries.

CLINICS CARE POINTS

- The prognosis after SCI is most dependent on the degree of residual neurologic motor function after injury. Motor incomplete patients show the highest propensity for significant functional improvement.

- Improvement in AIS grade does not correlate with functional improvement.

- Future studies from registries and "=big data will continue to improve our understanding of the natural history of SCI.

DISCLOSURE

The authors do not report conflicts of interest concerning the materials and methods used in this study or the findings specified in this paper.

REFERENCES

1. Batchelor PE, Tan S, Wills TE, et al. Comparison of inflammation in the brain and spinal cord following mechanical injury. J Neurotrauma 2008;25:1217–25.
2. Tsolinas RE, Burke JF, DiGrgio AM, et al. Transforming research and clinical knowledge in spinal cord injury (TRACK-SCI): an overview of initial enrollment and demographics. Neurosurg Focus 2020;48(5):E6.
3. Spinal Cord Injury Facts and Figures at a Glance. J Spinal Cord Med 2014;37(3):355–6.
4. Burns S, Biering-Sørensen F, Donovan W, et al. International standards for neurological classification of spinal cord injury, revised 2011. Top Spinal Cord Inj Rehabil 2012;18(1):85–99.
5. El Tecle NE, Dahdaleh NS, Bydon M, et al. The natural history of complete spinal cord injury: a pooled analysis of 1162 patients and a meta-analysis of modern data. J Neurosurg Spine 2018;28(4): 436–43.
6. Tator CH. Review of treatment trials in human spinal cord injury: issues, difficulties, and recommendations. Neurosurgery 2006;59(5):957–82.
7. Burns AS, Marino RJ, Flanders AE, et al. Clinical diagnosis and prognosis following spinal cord injury. Handb Clin Neurol 2012;109:47–62.
8. Waters RL, Adkins R, Yakura J, et al. Functional and neurologic recovery following acute SCI. J Spinal Cord Med 1998;21:195–9.
9. Scivoletto G, Tamburella F, Laurenza L, et al. Who is going to walk? A review of the factors influencing walking recovery after spinal cord injury. Front Hum Neurosci 2014;8(MAR):141.
10. Marino RJ, Ditunno JF, Donovan WH, et al. Neurologic recovery after traumatic spinal cord injury: data from the model spinal cord injury systems. Arch Phys Med Rehabil 1999;80(11):1391–6.
11. Fawcett JW, Curt A, Steeves JD, et al. Guidelines for the conduct of clinical trials for spinal cord injury as developed by the ICCP panel: spontaneous recovery after spinal cord injury and statistical power needed for therapeutic clinical trials. Spinal Cord 2007;45(3):190–205.
12. Burke JF, Yue JK, Ngwenya LB, et al. Ultra-Early (<12 Hours) surgery correlates with higher rate of American Spinal Injury Association impairment scale conversion after cervical spinal cord injury. Neurosurgery 2019;85(2):199–203.
13. Scivoletto G, Morganti B, Molinari M. Neurologic recovery of spinal cord injury patients in Italy. Arch Phys Med Rehabil 2004;85(3):485–9.
14. Waters RL, Yakura JS, Adkins RH, et al. Recovery following complete paraplegia. Arch Phys Med Rehabil 1992;73(9):784–9.
15. Waters RL, Adkins RH, Yakura JS, et al. Motor and sensory recovery following complete tetraplegia. Arch Phys Med Rehabil 1993;74(3):242–7.
16. Kirshblum S, Millis S, McKinley W, et al. Late neurologic recovery after traumatic spinal cord injury. Arch Phys Med Rehabil 2004;85(11):1811–7.
17. Burns AS, Lee BS, Ditunno JF, et al. Patient selection for clinical trials: the reliability of the early spinal cord injury examination. J Neurotrauma 2003;20(5): 477–82.
18. Bracken MB, Shepard MJ, Collins WF, et al. A randomized, controlled trial of methylprednisolone or naloxone in the treatment of acute spinal-cord injury. N Engl J Med 1990;322(20): 1405–11.
19. Bracken MB, Shepard MJ, Collins WF, et al. Methylprednisolone or naloxone treatment after acute spinal cord injury: 1-year follow-up data: results of the second National Acute Spinal Cord Injury Study. J Neurosurg 1992;76(1):23–31.
20. Khorasanizadeh MH, Yousefifard M, Eskian M, et al. Neurological recovery following traumatic spinal cord injury: a systematic review and meta-analysis. J Neurosurg Spine 2019;30(5):683–99.
21. Medana IM, Esiri MM. Axonal damage: a key predictor of outcome in human CNS diseases. Brain 2003; 126(3):515–30.
22. Rowland JW, Hawryluk GWJ, Kwon B, et al. Current status of acute spinal cord injury pathophysiology and emerging therapies: promise on the horizon. Neurosurg Focus 2008;25(5):E2.
23. Curt A, Van Hedel HJA, Klaus D, et al. Recovery from a spinal cord injury: significance of compensation, neural plasticity, and repair. J Neurotrauma 2008;25:677–85.
24. Waters RL, Adkins RH, Yakura JS, et al. Motor and sensory recovery following incomplete paraplegia. Arch Phys Med Rehabil 1994;75(1):67–72.
25. Waters RL, Adkins RH, Yakura JS, et al. Motor and sensory recovery following incomplete tetraplegia. Arch Phys Med Rehabil 1994;75(3):306–11.
26. O'Shea TM, Burda JE, Sofroniew MV. Cell biology of spinal cord injury and repair. J Clin Invest 2017; 127(9):3259–70.
27. Ditunno PL, Patrick M, Stineman M, et al. Who wants to walk? Preferences for recovery after SCI: a longitudinal and cross-sectional study. Spinal Cord 2008; 46(7):500–6.
28. Van Middendorp JJ, Hosman AJF, Pouw MH, et al. ASIA impairment scale conversion in traumatic SCI: is it related with the ability to walk? A descriptive comparison with functional ambulation outcome measures in 273 patients. Spinal Cord 2009;47(7): 555–60.

29. Ditunno JF, Scivoletto G, Patrick M, et al. Validation of the walking index for spinal cord injury in a US and European clinical population. Spinal Cord 2008;46(3):181–8.

30. Jakob W, Wirz M, van Hedel HJA, et al. Difficulty of Elderly SCI Subjects to Translate Motor Recovery—"Body Function"—into Daily Living Activities. J Neurotrauma 2009;26(11):2037–44.

31. Wagner FB, Mignardot J-B, Le Goff-Mignardot CG, et al. Targeted neurotechnology restores walking in humans with spinal cord injury. Nature 2018; 563(7729):65–71.

32. Harkema S, Gerasimenko Y, Hodes J, et al. Effect of epidural stimulation of the lumbosacral spinal cord on voluntary movement, standing, and assisted stepping after motor complete paraplegia: a case study. Lancet 2011;377(9781):1938–47.

33. Angeli CA, Boakye M, Morton RA, et al. Recovery of over-ground walking after chronic motor complete spinal cord injury. N Engl J Med 2018;379(13): 1244–50.

34. Gill ML, Grahn PJ, Calvert JS, et al. Neuromodulation of lumbosacral spinal networks enables independent stepping after complete paraplegia. Nat Med 2018;24(11):1677–82.

35. Dimitrijevic MR, Gerasimenko Y, Pinter MM. Evidence for a spinal central pattern generator in humans. Ann NY Acad Sci 1998;860(1 NEURONAL MECH):360–76.

36. Illis LS. Is there a central pattern generator in man? Spinal Cord 1995;33(5):239–40.

37. Harkema SJ, Hurley SL, Patel UK, et al. Human lumbosacral spinal cord interprets loading during stepping. J Neurophysiol 1997;77(2):797–811.

38. Barbeau H, Blunt R. A novel interactive locomotor approach using body weight support to retrain gait in spastic paretic subjects. In: Wernig A, editor. Plasticity of motoneuronal connections. 1991. p. 461–74.

39. Capogrosso M, Milekovic T, Borton D, et al. A brain–spine interface alleviating gait deficits after spinal cord injury in primates. Nature 2016;539(7628): 284–8.

40. Biering-Sørensen F, Alai S, Anderson K, et al. Common data elements for spinal cord injury clinical research: a national institute for neurological disorders and stroke project. Spinal Cord 2015;53(4): 265–77.

41. Yue JK, Hemmerle DD, Winkler EA, et al. Clinical implementation of novel spinal cord perfusion pressure protocol in acute traumatic spinal cord injury at U.S. level I trauma center: TRACK-SCI Study. World Neurosurg 2020;133:e391–6.

42. Talbott JF, Whetstone WD, Readdy WJ, et al. The Brain and Spinal Injury Center score: a novel, simple, and reproducible method for assessing the severity of acute cervical spinal cord injury with axial T2-weighted MRI findings. J Neurosurg Spine 2015; 23(4):495–504.

Diagnostic Imaging in Spinal Cord Injury

Saman Shabani, MD[a], Briana P. Meyer, BS[a,b], Matthew D. Budde, PhD[a,c], Marjorie C. Wang, MD, MPH[a,*]

KEYWORDS

- Diagnostic • Imaging • MRI • Diffusion tensor imaging • Spinal cord injury • Spinal trauma

KEY POINTS

- Spinal imaging, specifically computed tomography (CT) and MRI, is essential to the diagnosis of spinal trauma and spinal cord injury.
- Multidetector CT is the initial imaging modality for evaluation of spinal trauma with axial acquisition and multiplanar reconstructions of the entire spine.
- MRI provides information about soft tissue, disk, ligaments, and spinal cord, and is complementary to CT in evaluation of spinal trauma.
- Diffusion tensor imaging (DTI) provides information about microscopic structure of the spinal cord but clinical use in the acute setting is limited because of variations in scanner performance and postprocessing requirements. Recent advances may help improve the clinical applicability of DTI.
- Perfusion MRI and intraoperative contrast-enhanced ultrasonography are promising new techniques that may prove useful adjuncts to current imaging modalities.

INTRODUCTION

Diagnostic imaging is invaluable in the evaluation of patients with suspected spinal cord injury (SCI) in the acute setting. Imaging-based classification schemes may be used to describe the extent and severity of spinal cord damage. Imaging characteristics are also associated with post-SCI outcomes and may provide potential biomarkers of injury. This article discusses the role of imaging in the diagnosis of patients with SCI and highlights recent developments and promising new techniques and their potential clinical impacts.

IMAGING IN ACUTE SPINAL CORD INJURY DIAGNOSIS
Radiographs and Computed Tomography

In the past, radiography (plain radiograph) was the initial imaging modality in evaluation of spinal trauma. However, radiography has limited sensitivity (30%–60%) for the detection of bony and ligamentous injuries in patients for whom there is a high suspicion of spinal injury.[1] Diaz and colleagues[2] evaluated 116 patients with 172 fractures and found that 52% of cervical spine injuries were missed on plain films compared with computed tomography (CT), of which 17.5% were deemed unstable. Platzer and colleagues[3] also found CT to be more sensitive than cross-table lateral radiographs in patients with cervical spine fractures; CT had sensitivity of 97% to 100% in identifying cervical spine fractures compared with cross-table lateral radiographs, which had sensitivity of only 63%. In a prospective study by Widder and colleagues,[4] the sensitivity, specificity, and accuracy of plain films compared with CT scans were 39%, 98%, and 88%, respectively in the cervical spine. In studies that compared both radiographs and CT in thoracolumbar trauma, CT was associated with sensitivity ranging from 78.1% to

[a] Department of Neurosurgery, Medical College of Wisconsin, 8701 West Watertown Plank Road, Wauwatosa, WI 53226, USA; [b] Department of Biophysics, Medical College of Wisconsin, Wauwatosa, WI, USA; [c] Clement J Zablocki Veteran's Affairs Medical Center, Milwaukee, WI, USA
* Corresponding author.
E-mail address: marjorie.wang@gmail.com

Neurosurg Clin N Am 32 (2021) 323–331
https://doi.org/10.1016/j.nec.2021.03.004
1042-3680/21/© 2021 Elsevier Inc. All rights reserved.

100%, whereas plain radiographs had sensitivity ranging from 32% to 74%.[5]

At present, CT is the preferred imaging modality for evaluation of spinal trauma, recommended by multiple societies and published guidelines (American College of Radiology,[6] American Association of Neurological Surgeons/Congress of Neurological Surgeons[7]; Advanced Trauma Life Support; Spinal Cord Trauma). In addition to providing detailed bony anatomy, CT findings can indicate significant soft tissue abnormalities based on pattern of injury and biomechanical principles. CT findings suggestive of ligamentous injury include prevertebral hematoma, spondylolisthesis, asymmetric disk space widening, facet joint widening or dislocations, angulation, and interspinous space widening.

Several studies have evaluated the additive value of MRI to CT scans in evaluating soft tissue injuries after spinal trauma. Hogan and colleagues[8] evaluated obtunded patients with both CT and cervical MRI. All subjects had a normal CT. Compared with MRI, which was performed a mean of 9 days after injury, CT had a negative predictive value of 98.8% for ligamentous injury and 100% for unstable cervical spine injury. Alhilali and Fakhran[9] compared CT and MRI completed within 7 days of trauma, to assess anterior cervical diskoligamentous injuries. Subjective assessment of disk space widening on CT yielded poor sensitivity (16%; 95% confidence interval, 10.5%, 24.3%). However, measurement of an intervertebral disk angle greater than 2 standard deviations from the average of the remaining disks provided a sensitivity of 72.1% (95% confidence interval, 63.2%, 79.7%) and specificity of 100% (95% confidence interval, 99.6%, 100%) for the detection of anterior cervical diskoligamentous injury. The investigators discuss that calculating a standard deviation in a clinical setting is impractical and suggest that other measurements, such as an intradiskal angle of 13° or more, might be a substitute for calculation, with an increase in false-positive results.[9] MRI is insensitive to some spinal fractures, especially those involving posterior elements,[10] but may reveal acute compressive marrow edema and thereby complement CT findings when chronicity is indeterminate. However, the presence and degree of edema vary; fractures without compression or fractures with only distraction do not reliably generate marrow edema and can lead to a false-negative study or miss the acuity of a fracture.[10]

At present, the American College of Radiography recommends limited use of plain radiographs, restricted mainly to settings in which there is a low suspicion of SCI or where CT is not possible.[6] If CT is not available, plain radiographic films from the occiput to T1, including lateral, anteroposterior (AP), and open-mouth odontoid views, should be obtained.[11] Two criteria are commonly used to help in decision making for cervical spine imaging in patients with trauma. These are the Canadian Cervical Spine rule and National Emergency X-radiography Utilization Study (NEXUS). Per NEXUS criteria,[12] cervical spine radiography is not indicated for patients who meet the following criteria:

1. No posterior midline cervical spine tenderness
2. No evidence of intoxication
3. A normal level of alertness
4. No focal neurologic deficit
5. No painful distracting injuries

Flexion-extension radiographs

Flexion-extension radiographs may be used to rule out ligamentous injury to the spine in patients with negative or nondiagnostic radiographs.[13] These views may be obtained in patients with persistent pain or tenderness in the presence of a negative CT scan. However, after acute injury to the neck, the presence of muscle spasm can result in a limited examination, and unstable ligamentous injuries may be masked by inadequate flexion and extension, considered to be greater than 30° of motion from the neutral cervical spine position.[13]

Computed Tomography Angiogram

Blunt cerebrovascular injuries may be identified in up to 1% of patients with blunt traumatic injuries, most commonly after motor vehicle crashes (80%).[1] Fractures of the craniocervical junction and foramen transversarium, vertebral body dislocations, and severe hyperextension or flexion injuries are indications for obtaining CT angiograms.[14] The Biffl classification is often used to grade the degree of blunt cerebrovascular injury in blunt traumas, and is associated with risk of stroke.[15]

MRI in Spinal Cord Injury

MRI is the gold standard imaging modality for the evaluation of the spinal cord in the acute setting. Recommended MRI sequences for spinal cord trauma include sagittal fast spin-echo (FSE), axial and sagittal T1-weighted imaging, axial and sagittal FSE T2-weighted imaging, sagittal T2-weighted fat-suppressed imaging (**Fig. 1**), and axial T2*-weighted gradient echo imaging (**Table 1**). Some variability in recommended MRI sequences may depend on the clinical presentation or magnetic resonance (MR) scanner capabilities.

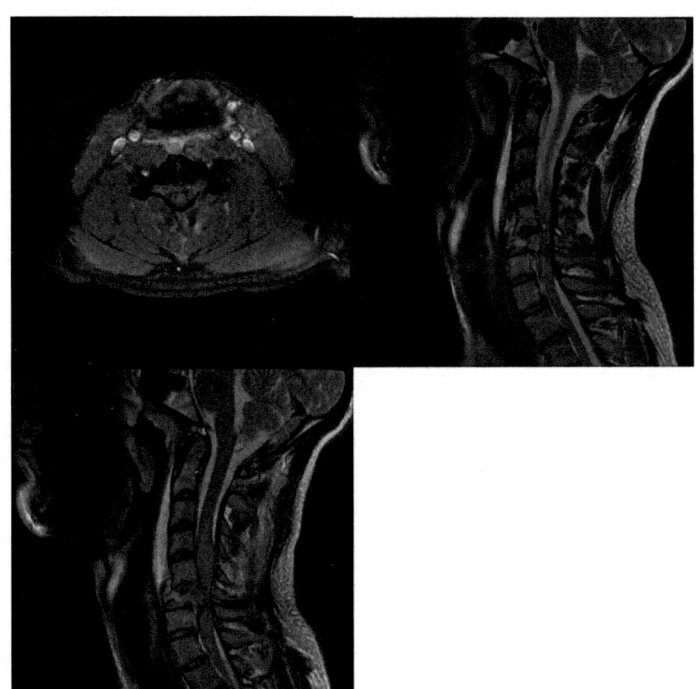

Fig. 1. Axial (*top left*) and sagittal (*top right and bottom left*) views of C6 burst fracture with retropulsion into the canal. The gradient recalled echo axial view shows multiple areas of microhemorrhage in the spinal cord. The T2 sagittal views show T2 hyperintensity as well as area of microhemorrhage within the cord.

Conventional MRI

Conventional MRI provides valuable information about spinal cord compression, ligamentous instability, and disk herniation, as well as intramedullary damage such as edema and hemorrhage.[16] Findings on MRI that raise the suspicion for injury to the ligamentous structures include the presence of a gap or an increased signal in the ligament or the surrounding structures (**Fig. 2**). High sensitivity to intramedullary disorder makes T2-weighted imaging the most used sequence in acute SCI, with both axial and sagittal views providing useful information for injury characterization.[16,17] T2-weighted MRI is sensitive to the paramagnetic effects of iron present in blood products, which results in hypointense areas indicating intramedullary hemorrhage.[16,18,19] In addition to T2-weighted sequences, T2*-weighted gradient echo and susceptibility-weighted imaging sequences are also used for detection of intramedullary hemorrhage.[20] Further, T2-weighted imaging can provide information regarding the edema.[21,22]

Conventional MRI and neurologic recovery

In addition to the clinical examination, T1-weighted and T2-weighted MRI characteristics have been used to define the extent of the injury in patients with SCI and to create classification schemes that are associated with the severity of

Table 1
Commonly used MRI sequences for evaluation of the spinal cord

MRI Sequence	Evaluation
T1-weighted imaging	Anatomy, hypointense marrow edema in acute fracture, isointense to hyperintense epidural hemorrhage
T2-weighted imaging	SCI, ligamentous injury, disk herniation; marrow edema may be masked by unsuppressed fat
STIR	SCI, ligamentous injury, disk herniation, marrow edema
T2*-weighted (gradient echo)	Intramedullary hemorrhage, epidural collections

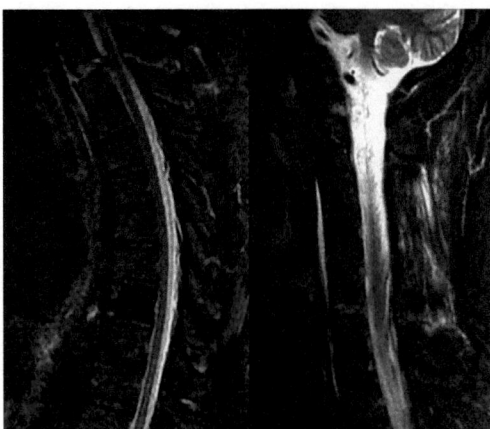

Fig. 2. Sagittal short tau inversion recovery (STIR) view of thoracic (*left*) and cervical (*right*) spine MRI. There is an increase in STIR signal across the T1/2 disk as well as the disk at C5/6 with involvement of the posterior elements.

the injury and neurologic outcome (**Table 2**). Kulkarni and colleagues[23] found spinal cord hemorrhage, edema, and swelling to be associated with SCI. In this classification system, hemorrhage was seen in more severe deficits, whereas edema was seen in patients with milder deficits.[23] Schaefer and colleagues[24] noted that hemorrhage (type 1 pattern) and edema spanning multiple vertebral segments (type 2 pattern) was associated with more severe deficits. In another study, Flanders and colleagues[25] found the presence of hemorrhage was predictive for a complete neurologic injury, whereas the length of spinal cord showing edema correlated with the severity of initial deficits. Another study by this group also showed hemorrhage and longer segments of edema correlated with poor functional recovery.[26]

In a prospective analysis, Boldin and colleagues[27] noted that hemorrhagic lesions of less than 4 mm were associated with incomplete SCI and neurologic recovery. However, a hemorrhage greater than 10 mm was often associated with complete SCI,[28] particularly if it was in the cervical spinal cord.[25] In addition, Talbot and colleagues[30] developed a novel 5-point ordinal MRI score (Brain and Spinal Injury Center [BASIC] score) based on the axial images at the epicenter of SCI[17,29,30] and the amount of hemorrhage and edema. However, the most sensitive predictor of long-term prognosis remains the neurologic severity of SCI on initial examination, with or without sacral sparing.[31,32] There are limitations with this too, as Kirshblum and colleagues[32] describe, including factors such as a patient's ability to cooperate with the examination and variability in the assessor's

Table 2 MRI-based classification schemes	
Kulkarni et al.[33] (1988) MRI Patterns for Prognosticating Acute SCI	
Pattern 1	Hemorrhage in the cord
Pattern 2	Edema in the cord
Pattern 3	Mixture of hemorrhage and edema in the cord
Bondurant et al.[34] (1990) Classification Scheme for Prognostication of Acute SCI	
Pattern 1	Normal MRI signal
Pattern 2	Single-level edema
Pattern 3	Multilevel edema
Pattern 4	Mixed hemorrhage and edema
Schaefer et al.[24] (1989) Types of MRI Findings Associated with Acute SCI	
Type 1	Central intramedullary cord hemorrhage
Type 2	T2-hyperintense contusion extending longitudinally >1 vertebral body
Type 3	T2-hyperintense contusion was confined to a single vertebral body
Type 4	No evidence of SCI on MRI
The BASIC Score for Classifying Acute SCIs Using Axial T2-weighted Imaging	
BASIC 0	No intramedullary cord signal abnormality
BASIC 1	Intramedullary T2 hyperintensity confined to central gray matter
BASIC 2	Intramedullary T2 hyperintensity involves both gray and white matter but does not cover the entire transverse extent of the spinal cord
BASIC 3	Intramedullary T2 hyperintensity covers the entire transverse extent of the spinal cord
BASIC 4	Intramedullary T2 hyperintensity covers the entire transverse extent of the spinal cord plus T2-hypointense foci

Abbreviation: BASIC, Brain and Spinal Injury Center.

training and experience. Other factors that may also contribute to heterogeneity in outcome include timing of the assessments.

Over time, T2-weighted imaging characteristics change after traumatic SCI. In the acute setting,

T2-weighted imaging shows edema as well as hemorrhage.[35] In the subacute setting, there is expansion of the lesion.[22,36] In the chronic setting, atrophy and cyst formation usually occur within the first month after injury.[37] Small tissue bridges may be seen around the posttraumatic cyst on T2-weighted imaging scans and can indicate a better prognosis for long-term functional recovery.[37] Huber and colleagues[37] noted that presence and size of midsagittal tissue bridges and smaller posttraumatic lesions at 1 month were associated with better neurologic recovery at 1-year follow-up.

T2-weighted imaging is not very specific to the underlying pathophysiology behind SCI. High T2 signal can be seen in the spinal cord from edema, hemorrhage, inflammation, demyelination, cyst cavitation, or the development of myelomalacia.[30] Depending on the timing of MRI after injury, the T2-weighted imaging findings are different and variable across patients.[21] This difference has led to development of quantitative imaging modalities that better show the microstructural changes that occur in SCI.

Diffusion-Weighted Imaging

One of the most commonly used quantitative imaging modalities is diffusion-weighted MRI (DWI). Diffusion-weighted sequences are increasingly incorporated into standard MR protocols to better delineate microstructural changes in the hope of identifying biomarkers linked to clinical outcome.[38] This technique is still in the research phase and is not routinely used to guide clinical care. Diffusion tensor imaging (DTI) is an extension of DWI that quantifies the three-dimensional characteristics of water diffusion and can be used to infer microstructure, although water diffusion is an indirect measure of cord integrity and disorder (**Fig. 3**). The 2 most frequently used metrics are fractional anisotropy (FA) and mean diffusivity (MD) or apparent diffusion coefficient (ADC). Other metrics commonly studied include axial diffusivity (AD) or longitudinal ADC (lADC), and radial diffusivity (RD) or transverse ADC (tADC). Briefly, FA is a measure of the extent of asymmetry in the diffusion of water molecules within the spinal cord, MD represents the average diffusion rate of the water molecules irrespective of the direction, AD evaluates the diffusion of water molecules in the spinal cord along the rostrocaudal direction, and RD highlights the diffusion of[10] water molecules perpendicular to the rostrocaudal direction.

Prior studies have consistently shown that FA is decreased, and MD is increased, in patients with SCI compared with controls.[39–43] Shabani and

colleagues[44] evaluated the diagnostic and prognostic value of DTI in both cervical and thoracic SCI. In patients with cervical SCI, FA in the high cervical (C1-C2) correlated significantly with injury severity and neurologic recovery 1-year after injury. However, in patients with thoracic SCI, no significant correlation was seen between FA and injury severity at 1-year follow-up.[44] The distance between the measurement site for FA (C1-C2) and the location of the injury in thoracic spine may contribute to this finding.[44] Poplawski and colleagues[45] found significant reductions in FA and increases in MD and RD proximal to the injury site (within 1 level above and below epicenter). DTI indices measured immediately rostral to the anatomic level of injury consistently showed better correlation with the extent of injury and accuracy in predicting neurologic recovery at 6 months than indices measured at the epicenter. FA and RD measured 1 level rostral to the injury site had the best sensitivity and specificity for predicting the severity of injury. However, MD offered the best prediction of neurologic recovery.[45]

Diffusion tensor imaging in cervical myelopathy

DTI has been extensively studied in patients with cervical spondylotic myelopathy (CSM), which, because of underlying spinal cord compression, has certain characteristics in common with SCI. In a cohort of 27 patients with CSM, Vedantam and colleagues[46] found the mean FA at the level

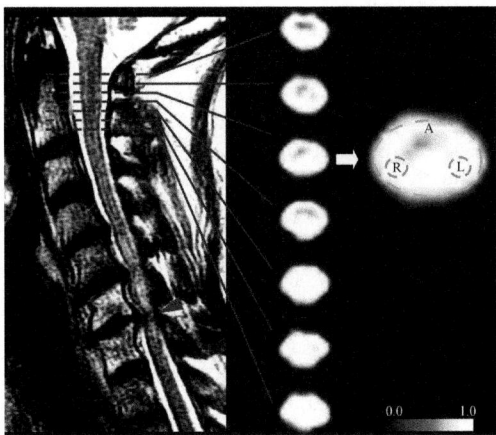

Fig. 3. Sagittal cervical spine T2-weighted image showing 7 axial fractional anisotropy maps through the high cervical cord (*red dotted line*). Solid arrowhead shows the injury site at the C6-C7 intervertebral disk level. A single fractional anisotropy map is magnified to show the whole cord regions of interest (*green*) and the regions of interest for the corticospinal tracts (*blue*). A, anterior; L, left; R, right.

of maximal compression was lower compared with the mean FA at the high cervical cord (C1-C2). FA correlated both with the preoperative modified Japanese Orthopedic Association (mJOA) score and the change in mJOA score before surgery and at follow-up 3 months after surgery.[46–48] Rao and colleagues[49] performed a large prospective study of surgically treated patients with CSM with the goal of determining whether FA can be used as a biomarker for defining who will benefit from surgical intervention. Changes in mJOA score before and after surgery were obtained at follow-up at 3, 6, 12, and 24 months. The investigators determined that a preoperative FA value of less than 0.55 could be used as a cut-off value in selecting patients with CSM who stood to benefit from surgical intervention by having greatest improvements in mJOA scores following decompressive surgery.[49] Shabani and colleagues[47] conducted a prospective study on surgically treated patients with CSM to determine whether FA values or normalized T2 signal intensity was a better biomarker of disease severity and prognosis. The correlation between preoperative FA values, normalized T2 signal intensity, and the change in mJOA before and after surgery at 3, 6, 12, and 24 months was assessed. FA was more strongly correlated with change in mJOA score than normalized T2 signal intensity for predicting disease severity as well as long-term outcomes following surgery in patients with CSM.[47] FA may ultimately prove helpful in predicting the effect of surgery for patients with SCI as well.

Limitations in diffusion tensor imaging

Although DTI is a promising biomarker of SCI damage and prognosis, its clinical utility remains limited. In the past, low signal-to-noise ratio has limited image resolution, but wider adoption of 3-T and higher field strengths along with improvements in radiofrequency coils tailored to the spine continue to offer substantial gains in image quality. Spinal cord imaging has also typically suffered from artifact susceptibility arising from cardiac and respiratory motion, which can result in quantification errors of DTI parameters. Gating strategies may be used to reduce artifacts, but protocols differ by institution. Differences in post-processing techniques have also made it difficult to generalize DTI findings, and the added time and resources required for the post-processing may limit clinical use in the acute setting. Efforts to facilitate and standardize image acquisition and processing are in play and may help resolve some of these issues. For example, the Spinal Cord Toolbox is a free open-source toolkit with active developments to allow automatic quantitative analysis of spinal

cord MRI data in research settings.[50] Whether these advances will improve the utility of DTI in clinical diagnosis and prognosis remains to be further evaluated.

Recent advances in diffusion tensor imaging

Recent advances to overcome the limitations of DTI have also emerged. Notably, DTI is confounded by edema, which can mask damage to neurons. Skinner and colleagues[51,52] demonstrated a DWI technique in animal models termed double diffusion encoding or filtered DWI (fDWI) that reduces contamination from edema. Their method makes use of diffusion weighting to suppress signals from extracellular water such as edema and cerebrospinal fluid, minimizing their effect on DWI metrics. The result is better imaging contrast than DTI with strong correlation to functional outcomes in a rat model of SCI. Importantly, the technique has recently been shown to be compatible with current clinical DWI methods (ie, pulse sequences), requiring only minor modifications to the strength and direction of the applied diffusion directions specific to the spinal cord anatomy. Hence, widespread application across sites and institutions is possible. Efforts are ongoing to translate these methods into clinical use for patients with SCI.

PERFUSION IMAGING

Blood flow after traumatic SCI is disrupted because of physical damage to the microvasculature, neurogenic shock or hypovolemia, and dysregulation of the sympathetic nervous system following SCI, especially in the cervical spine.[53,54] Current clinical recommendations advocate hemodynamic management of patients with SCI,[55] but a non-invasive technique to monitor cord perfusion remains an unmet clinical need and an active area of research.

Perfusion MRI

Perfusion MRI is routine in the brain, but its application to the spinal cord is notably absent; there are no reports of perfusion MRI in patients with SCI. Dynamic susceptibility contrast (DSC) MRI, a gadolinium contrast technique, has recently been reported in cervical spondylosis with blood volume and oxygen extraction related to neurologic impairment.[56] However, only whole-cord metrics have been reported instead of perfusion maps. DSC imaging is challenged by susceptibly distortions and the small volume of tissue being imaged. A perfusion MRI method making use of endogenous contrast (without injection) called arterial spin labeling (ASL) has been reported in animal SCI with evidence of decreased blood flow following cervical and lumbar injury.[57] ASL has recently been further developed in rat SCI to reveal disrupted perfusion at the site of injury and the dynamics of cord perfusion and arterial supply. Further refinement of ASL in the spinal cord is needed for patient translation but represents a truly noninvasive method to monitor cord perfusion.

Intraoperative Imaging Methods

Intraoperative methods for perfusion imaging may be useful for surgical guidance, such as end points for decompression, or may provide crucial information to inform hemodynamic management in the intensive care unit. Khaing and colleagues[58] showed the utility of contrast-enhanced ultrasonography (CEUS) to identify regions of hypoperfusion, vascular damage, and decreased blood flow velocity following traumatic SCI in a rodent model. CEUS has also been reported useful in porcine acute SCI[59] and in patients with thoracic cord stenosis undergoing decompressive surgery.[60] Laser speckle contrast imaging is another intraoperative technique recently shown to be sensitive to spinal cord blood flow in acutely injured patients. Gallagher and colleagues[61] identified 3 distinct perfusion patterns after severe thoracic injury, suggesting a need for perfusion imaging to determine appropriate hemodynamic management in this heterogeneous population. Both intraoperative techniques provide high spatial and temporal resolution and, with clinical translation, may guide personalized interventions and therapy following SCI.

SUMMARY

In the evaluation of spinal trauma, diagnostic imaging, in conjunction with the neurologic examination, is of crucial importance. CT is currently the recommended first-line imaging modality because of its rapid acquisition and high sensitivity for osseous abnormalities. MRI provides complementary information about SCI as well as soft tissues. DTI provides microstructural information about the integrity of the axons and myelin sheaths, but its clinical use is limited by sensitivity to artifact, scanner variability, and the need for extensive postprocessing of images. Novel imaging techniques, such as double diffusion encoding, and perfusion studies may be better suited for the acute clinical setting and show promise in prognostication of outcome and monitoring therapeutic interventions.

CLINICS CARE POINTS

- In the setting of trauma, published decision aids may be used to guide clinical care for best practices in imaging, and specifically radiographs, to evaluate for spinal injuries.
- CT is the initial imaging modality of choice for evaluation of spinal trauma because of its rapid acquisition and ability to show osseous structural details.
- MRI should be obtained in settings of suspected SCI.
- DTI is of limited utility in the acute setting because of scanner variations and postprocessing requirements, but recent advances may mitigate these limitations. Newer imaging techniques hold promise for future clinical use.

ACKNOWLEDGMENTS

The authors wish to thank Mayank Kaushal, MD, MBA. Medical College of Wisconsin, Department of Neurosurgery for his contributions to this manuscript.

DISCLOSURE

The authors and Mayank Kaushal have nothing to disclose.

REFERENCES

1. Izzo R, Popolizio T, Balzano RF, et al. Imaging of cervical spine traumas. Eur J Radiol 2019;117:75–88.
2. Diaz JJ Jr, Gillman C, Morris JA Jr, et al. Are five-view plain films of the cervical spine unreliable? A prospective evaluation in blunt trauma patients with altered mental status. J Trauma 2003;55(4): 658–63 [discussion: 663–4].
3. Platzer P, Jaindl M, Thalhammer G, et al. Clearing the cervical spine in critically injured patients: a comprehensive C-spine protocol to avoid unnecessary delays in diagnosis. Eur Spine J 2006;15(12): 1801–10.
4. Widder S, Doig C, Burrowes P, et al. Prospective evaluation of computed tomographic scanning for the spinal clearance of obtunded trauma patients: preliminary results. J Trauma 2004;56(6):1179–84.
5. Wintermark M, Mouhsine E, Theumann N, et al. Thoracolumbar spine fractures in patients who have sustained severe trauma: depiction with multi-detector row CT. Radiology 2003;227(3):681–9.

6. Daffner RH, Hackney DB. ACR Appropriateness Criteria on suspected spine trauma. J Am Coll Radiol 2007;4(11):762–75.

7. Ryken TC, Hadley MN, Walters BC, et al. Radiographic assessment. Neurosurgery 2013;72(Suppl 2):54–72.

8. Hogan GJ, Mirvis SE, Shanmuganathan K, et al. Exclusion of unstable cervical spine injury in obtunded patients with blunt trauma: is MR imaging needed when multi-detector row CT findings are normal? Radiology 2005;237(1):106–13.

9. Alhilali LM, Fakhran S. Evaluation of the intervertebral disk angle for the assessment of anterior cervical diskoligamentous injury. AJNR Am J Neuroradiol 2013;34(12):2399–404.

10. Brinckman MA, Chau C, Ross JS. Marrow edema variability in acute spine fractures. Spine J 2015;15(3):454–60.

11. American College of S, Committee on T. Advanced trauma life support : student course manual2018.

12. Hoffman JR, Mower WR, Wolfson AB, et al. Validity of a set of clinical criteria to rule out injury to the cervical spine in patients with blunt trauma. National Emergency X-Radiography Utilization Study Group. N Engl J Med 2000;343(2):94–9.

13. Insko EK, Gracias VH, Gupta R, et al. Utility of flexion and extension radiographs of the cervical spine in the acute evaluation of blunt trauma. J Trauma 2002;53(3):426–9.

14. Anaya C, Munera F, Bloomer CW, et al. Screening multidetector computed tomography angiography in the evaluation on blunt neck injuries: an evidence-based approach. Semin Ultrasound CT MR 2009;30(3):205–14.

15. Biffl WL, Moore EE, Offner PJ, et al. Blunt carotid arterial injuries: implications of a new grading scale. J Trauma 1999;47(5):845–53.

16. Bozzo A, Marcoux J, Radhakrishna M, et al. The role of magnetic resonance imaging in the management of acute spinal cord injury. J Neurotrauma 2011;28(8):1401–11.

17. Haefeli J, Mabray MC, Whetstone WD, et al. Multivariate Analysis of MRI Biomarkers for Predicting Neurologic Impairment in Cervical Spinal Cord Injury. AJNR Am J Neuroradiol 2017;38(3):648–55.

18. Flanders AE, Spettell CM, Tartaglino LM, et al. Forecasting motor recovery after cervical spinal cord injury: value of MR imaging. Radiology 1996;201(3):649–55.

19. Hackney DB, Asato R, Joseph PM, et al. Hemorrhage and edema in acute spinal cord compression: demonstration by MR imaging. Radiology 1986;161(2):387–90.

20. Wang M, Dai Y, Han Y, et al. Susceptibility weighted imaging in detecting hemorrhage in acute cervical spinal cord injury. Magn Reson Imaging 2011;29(3):365–73.

21. Aarabi B, Sansur CA, Ibrahimi DM, et al. Intramedullary Lesion Length on Postoperative Magnetic Resonance Imaging is a Strong Predictor of ASIA Impairment Scale Grade Conversion Following Decompressive Surgery in Cervical Spinal Cord Injury. Neurosurgery 2017;80(4):610–20.

22. Le E, Aarabi B, Hersh DS, et al. Predictors of intramedullary lesion expansion rate on MR images of patients with subaxial spinal cord injury. J Neurosurg Spine 2015;22(6):611–21.

23. Kulkarni MV, McArdle CB, Kopanicky D, et al. Acute spinal cord injury: MR imaging at 1.5 T. Radiology 1987;164(3):837–43.

24. Schaefer DM, Flanders A, Northrup BE, et al. Magnetic resonance imaging of acute cervical spine trauma. Correlation with severity of neurologic injury. Spine (Phila Pa 1976) 1989;14(10):1090–5.

25. Flanders AE, Schaefer DM, Doan HT, et al. Acute cervical spine trauma: correlation of MR imaging findings with degree of neurologic deficit. Radiology 1990;177(1):25–33.

26. Flanders AE, Spettell CM, Friedman DP, et al. The relationship between the functional abilities of patients with cervical spinal cord injury and the severity of damage revealed by MR imaging. AJNR Am J Neuroradiol 1999;20(5):926–34.

27. Boldin C, Raith J, Fankhauser F, et al. Predicting neurologic recovery in cervical spinal cord injury with postoperative MR imaging. Spine (Phila Pa 1976) 2006;31(5):554–9.

28. Ramon S, Dominguez R, Ramirez L, et al. Clinical and magnetic resonance imaging correlation in acute spinal cord injury. Spinal Cord 1997;35(10):664–73.

29. Mabray MC, Talbott JF, Whetstone WD, et al. Multidimensional Analysis of Magnetic Resonance Imaging Predicts Early Impairment in Thoracic and Thoracolumbar Spinal Cord Injury. J Neurotrauma 2016;33(10):954–62.

30. Talbott JF, Whetstone WD, Readdy WJ, et al. The Brain and Spinal Injury Center score: a novel, simple, and reproducible method for assessing the severity of acute cervical spinal cord injury with axial T2-weighted MRI findings. J Neurosurg Spine 2015;23(4):495–504.

31. Kirshblum SC, O'Connor KC. Levels of spinal cord injury and predictors of neurologic recovery. Phys Med Rehabil Clin N Am 2000;11(1):1–27, vii.

32. Kirshblum S, Snider B, Eren F, et al. Characterizing natural recovery after traumatic spinal cord injury. J Neurotrauma 2021. https://doi.org/10.1089/neu.2020.7473.

33. Kulkarni MV, McArdle CB, Kopanicky D, et al. Acute spinal cord injury: MR imaging at 1.5 T. Radiology 1987;164(3):837–43.

34. Bondurant FJ, Cotler HB, Kulkarni MV, McArdle CB, Harris Jr J. Acute spinal cord injury. A study using physical examination and magnetic resonance imaging. Spine 1990;15(3):161–8.

35. Dhall SS, Haefeli J, Talbott JF, et al. Motor Evoked Potentials Correlate With Magnetic Resonance

Imaging and Early Recovery After Acute Spinal Cord Injury. Neurosurgery 2018;82(6):870–6.

36. Dalkilic T, Fallah N, Noonan VK, et al. Predicting Injury Severity and Neurological Recovery after Acute Cervical Spinal Cord Injury: A Comparison of Cerebrospinal Fluid and Magnetic Resonance Imaging Biomarkers. J Neurotrauma 2018;35(3):435–45.

37. Huber E, Lachappelle P, Sutter R, et al. Are midsagittal tissue bridges predictive of outcome after cervical spinal cord injury? Ann Neurol 2017;81(5):740–8.

38. Kaushal M, Shabani S, Budde M, et al. Diffusion Tensor Imaging in Acute Spinal Cord Injury: A Review of Animal and Human Studies. J Neurotrauma 2019;36(15):2279–86.

39. Cheran S, Shanmuganathan K, Zhuo J, et al. Correlation of MR diffusion tensor imaging parameters with ASIA motor scores in hemorrhagic and nonhemorrhagic acute spinal cord injury. J Neurotrauma 2011;28(9):1881–92.

40. Alizadeh M, Intintolo A, Middleton DM, et al. Reduced FOV diffusion tensor MR imaging and fiber tractography of pediatric cervical spinal cord injury. Spinal Cord 2017;55(3):314–20.

41. D'Souza MM, Choudhary A, Poonia M, et al. Diffusion tensor MR imaging in spinal cord injury. Injury 2017;48(4):880–4.

42. Shanmuganathan K, Gullapalli RP, Zhuo J, et al. Diffusion tensor MR imaging in cervical spine trauma. AJNR Am J Neuroradiol 2008;29(4):655–9.

43. Vedantam A, Eckardt G, Wang MC, et al. Clinical correlates of high cervical fractional anisotropy in acute cervical spinal cord injury. World Neurosurg 2015;83(5):824–8.

44. Shabani S, Kaushal M, Budde M, et al. Correlation of magnetic resonance diffusion tensor imaging parameters with American Spinal Injury Association score for prognostication and long-term outcomes. Neurosurg Focus 2019;46(3):E2.

45. Poplawski MM, Alizadeh M, Oleson CV, et al. Application of Diffusion Tensor Imaging in Forecasting Neurological Injury and Recovery after Human Cervical Spinal Cord Injury. J Neurotrauma 2019;36(21):3051–61.

46. Vedantam A, Rao A, Kurpad S, et al. Diffusion tensor imaging correlates with short-term myelopathy outcome in patients with cervical spondylotic myelopathy. World Neurosurg 2017;97:489–94.

47. Shabani S, Kaushal M, Budde M, et al. Comparison between quantitative measurements of diffusion tensor imaging and T2 signal intensity in a large series of cervical spondylotic myelopathy patients for assessment of disease severity and prognostication of recovery. J Neurosurg Spine 2019;131:473–9.

48. Shabani S, Kaushal M, Budde MD, et al. Diffusion tensor imaging in cervical spondylotic myelopathy: a review. J Neurosurg Spine 2020;1–8. https://doi.org/10.3171/2019.12.Spine191158.

49. Rao A, Soliman H, Kaushal M, et al. Diffusion tensor imaging in a large longitudinal series of patients with cervical spondylotic myelopathy correlated with long-term functional outcome. Neurosurgery 2018;83(4):753–60.

50. Cohen-Adad J, De Leener B, Benhamou M, et al. Spinal Cord Toolbox: an open-source framework for processing spinal cord MRI data. In Proceedings of the 20th Annual Meeting of OHBM, Hamburg, Germany, vol. 3633. 2014.

51. Skinner NP, Kurpad SN, Schmit BD, et al. Rapid in vivo detection of rat spinal cord injury with double-diffusion-encoded magnetic resonance spectroscopy. Magn Reson Med 2017;77(4):1639–49.

52. Skinner NP, Lee SY, Kurpad SN, et al. Filter-probe diffusion imaging improves spinal cord injury outcome prediction. Ann Neurol 2018;84(1):37–50.

53. Alizadeh A, Dyck SM, Karimi-Abdolrezaee S. Traumatic Spinal Cord Injury: An Overview of Pathophysiology, Models and Acute Injury Mechanisms. Front Neurol 2019;10:282.

54. Krassioukov A, Claydon VE. The clinical problems in cardiovascular control following spinal cord injury: an overview. Prog Brain Res 2006;152:223–9.

55. Walters BC, Hadley MN, Hurlbert RJ, et al. Guidelines for the management of acute cervical spine and spinal cord injuries: 2013 update. Neurosurgery 2013;60(CN_suppl_1):82–91.

56. Ellingson BM, Woodworth DC, Leu K, et al. Spinal Cord Perfusion MR Imaging Implicates Both Ischemia and Hypoxia in the Pathogenesis of Cervical Spondylosis. World Neurosurg 2019;128:e773–81.

57. Duhamel G, Callot V, Decherchi P, et al. Mouse lumbar and cervical spinal cord blood flow measurements by arterial spin labeling: sensitivity optimization and first application. Magn Reson Med 2009;62(2):430–9.

58. Khaing ZZ, Cates LN, Hyde J, et al. Contrast-enhanced ultrasound for assessment of local hemodynamic changes following a rodent contusion spinal cord injury. Mil Med 2020;185(Suppl 1):470–5.

59. Huang L, Lin X, Tang Y, et al. Quantitative assessment of spinal cord perfusion by using contrast-enhanced ultrasound in a porcine model with acute spinal cord contusion. Spinal Cord 2013;51(3):196–201.

60. Ling J, Jinrui W, Ligang C, et al. Evaluating perfusion of thoracic spinal cord blood using CEUS during thoracic spinal stenosis decompression surgery. Spinal Cord 2015;53(3):195–9.

61. Gallagher MJ, Hogg FRA, Zoumprouli A, et al. Spinal Cord Blood Flow in Patients with Acute Spinal Cord Injuries. J Neurotrauma 2019;36(6):919–29.

Spinal Cord Injury Clinical Classification Systems
What Is Available and a Proposed Alternative

Wyatt L. Ramey, MD[a],*, Jens R. Chapman, MD[b]

KEYWORDS

- Spinal cord injury • Neurotrauma • ASIA classification scale • Spine trauma • Spinal cord

KEY POINTS

- With the modern era of registries and "big data" routinely guiding clinical decision-making, it is important to have a universal, simple, and reliable means of documenting neurologic function in the spinal cord injured patient.
- Formal clinical assessment of spinal cord injury (SCI) needs a less cumbersome alternative to the American Spinal Injury Association that can be easily and widely administered.
- The proposed classification herein focuses on gross sensorimotor, sacral function below the injured level via an easy-to-use scoring system yielding grades 1 to 4 of injury severity.
- This classification system was designed for practicality in the clinical setting while maintaining granularity for research and scientific purposes.

INTRODUCTION

Acute traumatic spinal cord injury (SCI) is a serious neurologic condition with costly short-term and long-term impact for those affected, and the health care system in general. Physical, emotional, and financial repercussions are profound and a life-altering sentinel event for surviving patients and their families.[1] Epidemiologically speaking, SCI remains most prevalent in North America compared with other regions such as Western Europe and Australia and is presumed to be reflective of higher rates of violent crime and self-harm.[2,3] Outcome tools tracking neurologic function are therefore particularly relevant for North America.

Although there is a great abundance of work specifying the morphologic characteristics of spinal column fractures, there is much less literature classifying neurologic severity of injury and its prognosis, which lies at the center of clinical decision-making for SCI. The paucity of SCI classification systems in contrast to its relative importance is somewhat surprising, as neurologic impairment and prognosis routinely form the foundation for decision-making in clinical care and for data collection in registries and clinical trials.

Outcome scores and classification systems are widely used throughout clinical medicine. In everyday patient care they serve to facilitate efficient communication between medical professionals and guide management, whereas their use in research allows for long-term, accurate data collection as a tool to better determine efficacy of management strategies.[4] Relative to SCI care, classification systems and outcome tools first and foremost describe the severity of the acute injury, followed by the spinal cord level of injury and further attempts to prognosticate

[a] Department of Neurosurgery, Banner University of Arizona Medical Center – Tucson, PO Box 245070, 1501 North Campbell Avenue, Room 4303, Tucson, AZ 85724-5070, USA; [b] Department of Neurosurgery, Swedish Neuroscience Institute, 550 17th Avenue, Seattle, WA 98122, USA
* Corresponding author.
E-mail address: Wyattr12@email.arizona.edu

Neurosurg Clin N Am 32 (2021) 333–340
https://doi.org/10.1016/j.nec.2021.03.005
1042-3680/21/© 2021 Elsevier Inc. All rights reserved.

chances for neurologic function recovery. With the modern era of registries and "big data" now routinely guiding clinical decision-making, it is more important than ever to have a universal, simple, and reliable means of documenting neurologic function in the spinal cord injured patient. In this article the authors provide a review of SCI grading schemes, look at which best predict outcome and why, and integrate this into a proposal for SCI grading that will meet the needs of data repositories and clinical researchers over the next several decades.

Past and Current Classification Systems

Perhaps the most basic classification tool for SCI is the simple presence or absence of any neurologic deficit. This can be further differentiated into neurologically intact, incomplete, or complete SCI.[5] Frankel and colleagues[6] built on this by placing patients into 5 categories, A through E. Patients were categorized from severe complete sensorimotor SCI (A) to free of neurologic symptoms (E) (**Table 1**). Although proposed in the infancy SCI classifications, the Frankel grade was highly successful in its simplicity and clear interpretation and became a major tool going forward in diagnosing, predicting outcome in, and

treating multiple severities of SCI. Based purely on presenting neurologic symptoms, it acted as a guide to quickly and easily convey neurologic severity of the injury and ultimately the prognosis associated with such injuries. However, what the Frankel classification provides in its simplicity, it lacks in granularity, making it impractical in usage in modern research and data collection. Nonetheless, the Frankel classification provided a strong foundation on which future classifications of SCI were built.

It is generally accepted that most patients with acute SCIs, particularly those with incomplete SCI, are candidates for surgical intervention, as suggested by the Spine Trauma Study Group and reflected in the Thoracolumbar Injury Classification Score (TLICS).[7,8] TLICS is a numerical grading system used to guide surgical treatment of traumatic spine fractures. Points are assigned to each type of fracture morphology in the thoracolumbar spine, presence or absence of neurologic injury, and the integrity of the posterior ligamentous complex. A score of 0 to 3 suggests conservative (nonsurgical) management, greater than or equal to 5 suggests surgical management, and a score of 4 indicates surgeon's choice. Although TLICS primarily focuses on spinal column stability and integrity of the posterior

Table 1
Spinal cord injury classifications

	Brief Description	Strengths	Weaknesses
Frankel Classification	5-item scale ranging from complete SCI (A) to normal neurologic examination (E)	Easy to use across multiple disciplines; no computational requirements	Simplistic without numeric breakdown between grades; does not assess NLI
Functional Independence Measure (FIM)	18-item scale (each graded 1–7) assessing functional independence and ADLs	Provides detailed data on functional status and ADLs; provides longitudinal data for neurologic recovery	Performed by PT/OT; mostly limited to rehab or outpatient setting; does not assess NLI; includes cognition, which not always applicable
Spinal Cord Independence Measure (SCIM)	Numerical system (0–100) that assigns points on one's ability to perform specific tasks and ADLs	Provides detailed data on functional status and ADLs; provides longitudinal data for neurologic recovery; specific to spinal cord function	Requires PT, OT, and nurse to perform assessment; usually unable to perform acutely; does not assess NLI
Thoracolumbar Injury Classification Scale (TLICS)	Points system using fracture morphology, neurologic injury, and PLC integrity to assess need for surgery	Easy to use; integrates fracture morphology and neurologic status to guide treatment	Limited to thoracolumbar spine; does not provide prognosis for neurologic outcomes; does not assess NLI

Abbreviations: ADL, activities of daily living; NLI, neurologic level of injury; OT, occupational therapist; PLC, posterior ligamentous complex; PT, physical therapist.

ligamentous complex, it justifiably includes the Frankel philosophy of neurologic status as a function of "complete or incomplete" injury further broken down into spinal root, cord/conus medullaris, or cauda equina involvement.

Certainly, one of the strengths of this severity scale is integrating fracture morphology and acute neurologic status into one numeric value. Another strength is that TLICS can be easily and reliably calculated by most clinicians. Once a basic neurologic examination and appropriate imaging studies are complete (usually computed tomography and/or MR imaging), the spine surgery team can efficiently determine the TLICS score. Although TLICS can help assess the need for acute surgical intervention, it does not at all address the prognosis. Although it predicts which patients do poorly without surgery due to an unstable spinal column or posterior ligamentous complex, it does not have the computational means to predict neurologic outcome and recovery.

The Functional Independence Measure (FIM) is an 18-item scale measuring functionality and independence in activities of daily living. Each item is scaled on a 7-point scale with 7 representing complete independence and 1 requiring total assistance (unable to perform at least 25% of that particular task).[9] The FIM was developed through a collaboration between the American Academy of Physical Medicine and Rehabilitation and the American Congress of Rehabilitation Medicine and has been adopted by the SCI Model Systems for tracking and studying functional outcome after SCI.[10] Among different medical settings, providers, and types of patients, the FIM score demonstrates acceptable reliability and has proved utility particularly in the functional goals of physical rehabilitation research.[11] However, FIM requires rating of cognitive tasks rarely applicable to patients with SCI.

The Spinal Cord Independence Measure (SCIM) is a comprehensive tool that determines global independence following SCI by evaluating various tasks including self-care, respiratory and bowel/bladder control, and mobility of several types.[12,13] It was developed after FIM in part because results from the second North American Spinal Cord Injury Study (NASCIS II) failed to show any change in FIM, suggesting it to be insensitive to SCI. SCIM is a numerically graded 0 to 100 scale specific to general activities of daily living and independence. The strength of SCIM lies in its ability to track functional recovery specific to SCI in both rehabilitation and community settings.

Although FIM and SCIM generate granular, numerical data that can be used to gauge improvement after SCI, they lack practical application in the acute phase of SCI because both are built on outpatient tasks (stair management, outdoor mobility, transfer wheelchair-car, etc.).

Administration of these surveys also involves time-intensive examinations requiring multiple team members to perform. Physical therapists, occupational therapists, nurses, and rehabilitation specialists are suitably equipped for these assessments in the rehab setting, but they cannot be performed in acute care units. Furthermore, neither FIM nor SCIM provide insight into the neurologic level of injury (NLI) or objective residual neurologic function below the NLI. Hence there remains a need for an SCI evaluation tool that can consistently, uniformly, and efficiently assess function during acute inpatient care and yet remain relevant in short-term and long-term follow-up.

The American Spinal Injury Association grading system

When determining the degree of neurologic impairment in SCI, the most widely used system by far is the International Standards for Neurologic Classification of Spinal Cord Injury (ISNCSCI), also known as the American Spinal Injury Association (ASIA) score, which meticulously assesses motor and sensory function and overall impairment (**Table 2**).[14,15] The ASIA motor score examines each testable myotome from C5 to S1 on a standard scale of 0 to 5 strength, whereas the sensory examination determines appreciation of fine touch and pinprick in 28 dermatomes bilaterally from C2 to S5. Each of these components along with the ability to perform voluntary anal contraction and sense deep anal pressure are used to form the ASIA impairment scale (AIS) (see **Table 2**). Both the ASIA score and AIS grade should be documented as soon as possible following initial hospital presentation. The AIS grade, lettered from A to E, describes the overall severity of SCI and degree of remaining function and is directly associated with prognosis for neurologic recovery. An AIS score of A represents complete absence of any motor or sensory function below the NLI with loss of voluntary anal sphincter contraction. AIS grade D requires at least 50% of muscles below NLI to maintain greater than or equal to 4/5 strength. AIS E patients have normal motor and sensory function with no evidence of spinal cord impairment.

There are multiple studies in the scientific medical literature that correlate the prognosis of neurologic recovery in patients according to AIS grade. This remains a strength of the ASIA grading system by helping practitioners more predictably counsel patients and families on long-term outcome prospects.[16–21] For instance, less than

Table 2
The American Spinal Injury Association impairment scale

ASIA Motor Score	Calculated by grading each myotome 0–5 bilaterally; max score of 100
ASIA Sensory Score	Assesses presence/absence of light touch, pinprick sensation in each dermatome bilaterally
Voluntary Anal Function	Assesses presence/absence of voluntary anal contraction and deep anal sensation to determine sacral sparing
ASIA Impairment Scale (AIS)	
A	Complete SCI with no motor, sensory function below NLI; no sacral function
B	Motor complete, sensory incomplete SCI below NLI (including S4–5)
C	Motor incomplete SCI with >50% of myotomes below NLI <3 grade strength
D	Motor incomplete SCI with >50% of myotomes below NLI ≥3 grade strength
E	Normal motor and sensory function

5% of patients with ASIA A SCI will improve one or more AIS grades, with even fewer improving from a motor-complete to motor-incomplete status.[17] On the other hand, AIS B patients can convert to D in up to 40% of cases, whereas AIS C patients have a chance to convert to D in up to 80% of cases.[21] Over time the ASIA score and AIS grade have been shown to provide reliable, detailed data that can be used to track natural history, outcomes from various forms of treatment, and comparative analyses among differing types of patients with SCI.

The ISNCSCI/ASIA examination has been a major step forward in providing more specific and clinically relevant reproducible data for both clinical care and research endeavors. Interobserver and intraobserver reliability are high when assessing motor, light touch, and pinprick sensation scores and further suggest its utility in research protocols.[22,23] In addition, because of the high number of parameters and the specific degree to which each must be tested, the ASIA score offers a very complete picture of spinal neurologic impairment. Given its number of overall documented parameters, subanalyses are possible and usually plentifully represented in clinical studies. For example, not only is it possible to determine if patients with SCI will improve their overall AIS grade long term but it can also reliably track decline in NLI over time in simple and intuitively clear metrics.[17]

Formal ISNCSCI training is required for "certification" of investigators and their assistants to be able to perform ASIA assessments for the purposes of clinical trials and registries, even though the examination is widely delivered in everyday practice in most larger centers. Training requires sequential interaction with a certified instructor representing time and cost, highlighting the complexities of the examination and presenting a tangible barrier to universal application.

Although the AIS grade is an easily referenced tool that facilitates effective team communications detailing SCI severity and function, obtaining individual ASIA motor and sensory scores is a time-intensive and cumbersome assessment to perform, particularly in the setting of polytrauma or an intubated patient. The neurologic examination required to document ASIA status is exceedingly detailed requiring the examiner to assess every myotome and dermatome on each side of the body. This more than likely explains the heightened consistency and reproducibility of examinations beyond the 4-week period compared with baseline evaluations at the time of injury, as later examinations are conducted in a more controlled and focused setting in contrast to the environment of the acute management phase.[24] Because of the cumbersome nature of the ASIA examination, many patients with SCI cannot automatically undergo formal ASIA testing in the acute care phase and are therefore excluded from registries and large data sets that require a complete ASIA assessment.

An additional shortcoming of the ASIA assessment is the lack of attention to bowel, bladder, and sexual function despite the high importance of these outcomes in the SCI community. Each of these autonomic functions have a significant impact on the quality of life for people living with SCI; they also each have specific treatments with clear benefits.[25] A simple classification of bowel, bladder, and sexual functionality similarly is of high clinical relevance, but not adequately addressed by the presence or absence of sacral sensation, and conspicuously overlooked by the legacy classification systems.

A TOOL FOR NEXT-GENERATION SPINAL CORD INJURY ASSESSMENT

Where the ASIA scoring system succeeds in providing specific, detailed, granular data, it is simply a sum of its many parts and fails in providing an easy-to-use, applicable scoring system that all caregivers can easily administer and apply toward both patient care and clinical research. Providing detailed numeric data on each nerve root throughout the spinal column may be useful in terms of pure scientific data, but in addition to being cumbersome likely has little clinical relevance for predicting and monitoring recovery below the NLI. For example, a patient with a T8 AIS grade C SCI receives negligible value in a highly detailed motor assessment of each S1 nerve root.

With the shift of medical decision-making away from expensive randomized clinical trials toward research performed on big data warehouses, the prospect of ASIA-like assessments meeting the future needs of SCI investigators seems unlikely for all of the reasons outlined earlier. Yet even state-of-the-art surgery-specific data repositories such as National Surgical Quality Improvement Program and Quality Outcomes Database are poorly equipped to provide meaningful data on SCI. There is a growing need to embed SCI in big data with a twenty-first century solution. In 2010 van Middendorp and colleagues[26] presented their vision of key factors for an ideal spinal column injury classification. The investigators emphasized the preferable qualities maximizing suitability for everyday practical use by limiting the number of categories, thereby decreasing computational time necessary for arriving at alphanumerical grading. Similarly, each subcategory in the model system should also be characterized by increasing grades of severity represented by alphanumerical coding, thus improving intuitive clinical and research utility.

An ideal SCI scale should make use of many of the same parameters routinely collected by an experienced physician or nurse on initial assessment and during hospital stay. Over 60 years ago Long and colleagues[27] showed both neurologic and functional recovery strongly related to the NLI. Subsequently, hip flexion, hip extension, and hip abduction have been shown to correlate positively with ambulation after SCI, thus providing a

focused measure of important neurologic recovery and quality of life.[28,29] So although the NLI can provide immediate information guiding injury localization, treatment, and outcome, motor strength of the more proximal limb muscles complements day-to-day monitoring and prognostication.

The authors propose a 4-point motor score (0–3) below the NLI classified numerically into motor complete (0), motor major impaired,[1] motor minor impaired,[2] and normal[3] based on best muscle strength in any group for each limb *below the level of injury* (**Fig. 1**). Motor minor impaired is reflected in an incomplete SCI where there is preservation of clinically meaningful motor function in a limb below the NLI. Motor major impaired reflects no clinically meaningful motor function in any muscle groups of a given limb caudal to the NLI. "Clinically meaningful" neurologic function intuitively hinges on a minimum of antigravity strength in the best muscle group of a single limb. This circumvents needing to detail and calculate motor scores of 0 to 100 on each assessment, instead facilitating rapid and reliable SCI motor classification. This system also allows examiners to ignore attributes that arise out of missing or chronically dysfunctional limbs and accommodates cognitive impairments encountered in patients with comorbidities.

In a similar manner a sensory examination is simplified into one determination for each limb below the NLI (see **Fig. 1**). Sensory normal (2 points), sensory incomplete (1 point), and sensory complete (0 points) define the extent of sensory impairment based on best response in the limb to light touch appreciation—a universal and easy bedside test to perform. Importantly rectal tone, bulbocavernosus reflex, and perineal sensation are no longer required as part of an SCI score. Instead, independence (hand dexterity, ambulation, sphincter control) can be objectified in a non-acute care setting with the more detailed SCIM questionnaire.

A simplified evaluation of clinically meaningful motor and sensory function below the NLI will not only facilitate routine neurologic bedside monitoring in both intensive care unit and hospital ward settings, but will lend itself to become part of a core dataset for all patients admitted with a diagnosis of SCI. Simplification allows for granularity with an easy-to-use score that immediately conveys the severity of injury based on 2-limb (thoracolumbar injuries) or 4-limb (cervical injuries) assessment in distinct contrast to a cumbersome survey of every myotome and dermatome, sacral function, and zones of preservation. The scores generated by this simplified SCI score each indicate a specific degree of severity anticipated to directly reflect prognosis for return of neurologic

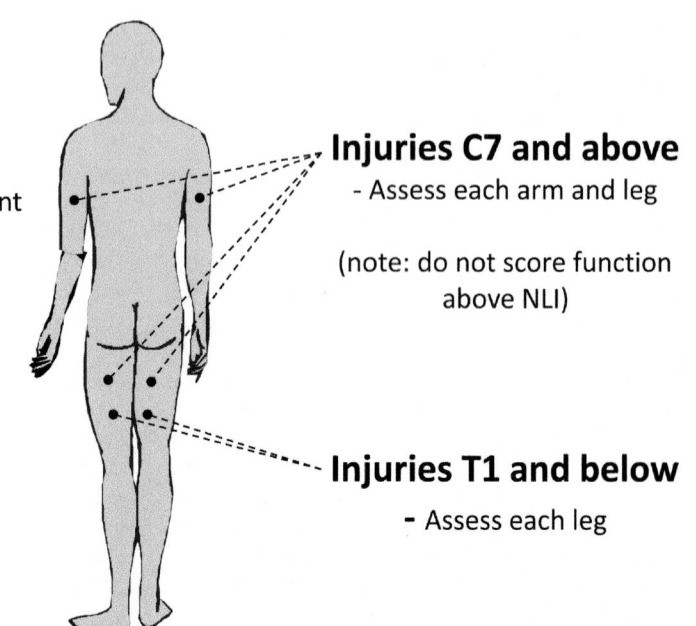

Motor
(Best motor group)
- 3 – normal
- 2 – antigravity movement
- 1 – non-antigravity movement
- 0 – no movement

Light Touch
(Best touch appreciation)
- 2 – normal
- 1 – present but altered
- 0 – absent

Injuries C7 and above
- Assess each arm and leg

(note: do not score function above NLI)

Injuries T1 and below
- Assess each leg

Fig. 1. Simplified neurologic assessment for SCI. Motor and sensory evaluations are completed on each limb below the neurologic level of injury (NLI). Motor scores are weighted heavier than sensory scores because they have more prognostic significance for functional recovery. A combined score of 10 (sum of motor and sensory for each limb) is normal for thoracic injuries, whereas a combined score of 20 is normal for cervical injuries at C7 and higher. Myotomes and dermatomes above the NLI should not be included in the assessment.

function, similar to AIS grade. Caregivers will not need special training or certification to receive "approval" in providing SCI evaluation nor will they need to include more invasive sphincter function as part of their routine examination.

Simplification of SCI scoring lends itself to App-based technology for rapid documentation and calculations on the spot. Such process improvements would also enhance examination compliance and analytical access, ideally generating systems rewards for any extra expenditures involved.

SUMMARY

The transformation of our world into a digitized "information age" mandates the need for useful, universal, granular data that can be practically obtained, effortlessly maintained, and quickly analyzed in large data repositories. The ASIA scoring system lacks simple "plug and go" parameters that are easily obtained by all qualified providers. Similar to burgeoning technological advances that have widespread, applicable functions relying on simplicity and ease-of-use, a contemporary method for classifying an entity as complex as SCI in the age of information must be simplified for the wave of "big data" that is on us now and guides our future. Turning the proverbial "big data" lakes into well organized "quantum"

data structures with ad hoc analytical functionality that does not sacrifice quality would be a profound step forwards for clinical SCI research. Modernizing our neurologic assessment of SCI can be regarded not only as an attractive option but also as a necessity to maximize enrollment, efficiency, and insight into improving SCI care. An alternative to the ASIA scale and AIS grading system such as the one we propose is needed to foster efficiency and maximize impact of neurologic data in this new age of informational technologies. Even though SCI is a complex traumatic and subsequent disease process with many contributing variables, simplifying our means of classification and prognostication applications will prove not only useful but also critical in going forward with future trials and registries.

CLINICS CARE POINTS

- SCI remains a challenging disease in terms of surgical decision-making and improving neurologic outcome.
- Quickly identifying and classifying varying severities of SCI is important in its short-term and long-term management.

- Outcome score and classification systems serve to facilitate efficient communication between clinicians and guide management, whereas their use in research allows for long-term, accurate data collection to better determine efficacy of management strategies.

DISCLOSURE

The authors have nothing to disclose.

REFERENCES

1. Ahuja CS, Wilson JR, Nori S, et al. Traumatic spinal cord injury. Nat Rev Dis Primers 2017;3(1):1–21.
2. Singh A, Tetreault L, Kalsi-Ryan S, et al. Global prevalence and incidence of traumatic spinal cord injury. Clin Epidemiol 2014;6:309.
3. Cripps RA, Lee BB, Wing P, et al. A global map for traumatic spinal cord injury epidemiology: towards a living data repository for injury prevention. Spinal Cord 2011;49(4):493–501.
4. Malterud K, Hollnagel H. The magic influence of classification systems in clinical practice. Scand J Prim Health Care 1997;15(1):5–6.
5. Burrell HL. I. Fracture of the spine: a summary of all the cases (244) which were treated at the Boston City Hospital from 1864 to 1905. Ann Surg 1905; 42(4):481.
6. Frankel HL, Hancock DO, Hyslop G, et al. The value of postural reduction in the initial management of closed injuries of the spine with paraplegia and tetraplegia. Spinal Cord 1969;7(3):179–92.
7. Lee JY, Vaccaro AR, Lim MR, et al. Thoracolumbar injury classification and severity score: a new paradigm for the treatment of thoracolumbar spine trauma. J Orthop Sci 2005;10(6):671.
8. Vaccaro AR, Zeiller SC, Hulbert RJ, et al. The thoracolumbar injury severity score: a proposed treatment algorithm. Clin Spine Surg 2005;18(3):209–15.
9. Hall KM, Cohen ME, Wright J, et al. Characteristics of the functional independence measure in traumatic spinal cord injury. Arch Phys Med Rehabil 1999;80(11):1471–6.
10. Granger CV, Hamilton BB, Keith RA, et al. Advances in functional assessment for medical rehabilitation. Top Geriatr Rehabil 1986;1(3):59–74.
11. Ottenbacher KJ, Hsu Y, Granger CV, et al. The reliability of the functional independence measure: a quantitative review. Arch Phys Med Rehabil 1996; 77(12):1226–32.
12. Catz A, Itzkovich M, Agranov E, et al. SCIM–spinal cord independence measure: a new disability scale for patients with spinal cord lesions. Spinal Cord 1997;35(12):850–6.
13. Itzkovich M, Gelernter I, Biering-Sorensen F, et al. The Spinal Cord Independence Measure (SCIM) version III: reliability and validity in a multi-center international study. Disabil Rehabil 2007;29(24):1926–33.
14. Kirshblum SC, Waring W, Biering-Sorensen F, et al. Reference for the 2011 revision of the international standards for neurological classification of spinal cord injury. J Spinal Cord Med 2011; 34(6):547–54.
15. American Spinal Injury Association. ISNCSCI worksheet. In: ASIA. 2000. Available at: http://asia-spinalinjury.org/information/downloads/. Accessed October 5, 2020.
16. Burns AS, Ditunno JF. Establishing prognosis and maximizing functional outcomes after spinal cord injury: a review of current and future directions in rehabilitation management. Spine (Phila Pa 1976) 2001;26(24 Suppl):S137–45.
17. Kirshblum S, Millis S, McKinley W, et al. Late neurologic recovery after traumatic spinal cord injury. Arch Phys Med Rehabil 2004;85(11):1811–7.
18. Wilson JR, Grossman RG, Frankowski RF, et al. A clinical prediction model for long-term functional outcome after traumatic spinal cord injury based on acute clinical and imaging factors. J Neurotrauma 2012;29(13):2263–71.
19. Coleman WP, Geisler FH. Injury severity as primary predictor of outcome in acute spinal cord injury: retrospective results from a large multicenter clinical trial. Spine J 2004;4(4):373–8.
20. van Middendorp JJ, Hosman AJ, Donders AR, et al. A clinical prediction rule for ambulation outcomes after traumatic spinal cord injury: a longitudinal cohort study. Lancet 2011;377(9770):1004–10.
21. Fawcett JW, Curt A, Steeves JD, et al. Guidelines for the conduct of clinical trials for spinal cord injury as developed by the ICCP panel: spontaneous recovery after spinal cord injury and statistical power needed for therapeutic clinical trials. Spinal Cord 2007;45(3):190–205.
22. Marino RJ, Jones L, Kirshblum S, et al. Reliability and repeatability of the motor and sensory examination of the international standards for neurological classification of spinal cord injury. J Spinal Cord Med 2008;31(2):166–70.
23. Savic G, Bergström EM, Frankel HL, et al. Inter-rater reliability of motor and sensory examinations performed according to American Spinal Injury Association standards. Spinal Cord 2007;45(6): 444–51.
24. Harrop JS, Maltenfort MG, Geisler FH, et al. Traumatic thoracic ASIA A examinations and potential for clinical trials. Spine 2009;34(23):2525–9.
25. Burns AS, Rivas DA, Ditunno JF. The management of neurogenic bladder and sexual dysfunction after spinal cord injury. Spine 2001;26(24S): S129–36.

26. van Middendorp JJ, Audigé L, Hanson B, et al. What should an ideal spinal injury classification system consist of? A methodological review and conceptual proposal for future classifications. Eur Spine J 2010; 19(8):1238–49.
27. Long C. Functional significance of spinal cord lesion level. Arch Phys Med Rehabil 1955;36:249–55.
28. Kim CM, Eng JJ, Whittaker MW. Level walking and ambulatory capacity in persons with incomplete spinal cord injury: relationship with muscle strength. Spinal Cord 2004;42(3):156–62.
29. Crozier KS, Cheng LL, Graziani V, et al. Spinal cord injury: prognosis for ambulation based on quadriceps recovery. Spinal Cord 1992;30(11):762–7.

Spinal Cord Injury Management on the Front Line

ABCs of Spinal Cord Injury Treatment Based on American Association of Neurological Surgeons/Congress of Neurological Surgeons Guidelines and Common Sense

Christopher Wilkerson, MD, Andrew T. Dailey, MD*

KEYWORDS

• Spinal cord injury • Stabilization • Airway management • Ventilatory support

KEY POINTS

- Monitoring patients with spinal cord injury in a surgical intensive care unit reduces mortality and can potentially improve outcome.
- Maintenance of mean arterial pressure >85 mmHg with volume replacement and pressors for 5-7 days improves spinal cord perfusion and likely improves neurological outcome in patients with spinal cord injury.
- Early reduction and stabilization of the patient with spinal cord injury through either open or closed methods provides the best chance of recovery.

INTRODUCTION

Spinal cord injury (SCI) affects approximately 54 per 1 million people annually in the United States.[1] Treatment strategies for this patient population focus on initial stabilization and early intervention. The cornerstones of early management are clinical assessment, characterization of the injury, medical optimization, and definitive surgical treatment, including surgical stabilization and/or decompression. This article discusses the important strategies in caring for patients with SCI that are supported with significant literature.

AIRWAY

Airway management must always come first as part of the initial Advanced Trauma Life Support

stabilization of patients with SCI, particularly for patients with cervical-level injuries. Como and colleagues[2] characterized the need for mechanical ventilation in patients with acute cervical SCI and neurologic deficits. They reported on 119 patients, 45 (37%) of whom had complete SCI. Twelve patients (27%) had injury levels from C1 to C4. Nineteen (42%) had a C5 injury, and 14 (31%) had an injury level of C6 or below. Eight of the patients with complete injury died, representing a mortality of 18%. All patients with complete SCI at the C5 level and above required intubation and an eventual tracheostomy. Of patients with a complete SCI at C6 or below, 79% required intubation; 50% of those went on to tracheostomy. As a result, the investigators strongly recommended early intubation be considered for patients with

Department of Neurosurgery, Clinical Neurosciences Center, University of Utah, 175 North Medical Drive East, Salt Lake City, UT 84132, USA
* Corresponding author.
E-mail address: neuropub@hsc.utah.edu

Neurosurg Clin N Am 32 (2021) 341–351
https://doi.org/10.1016/j.nec.2021.03.006
1042-3680/21/© 2021 Elsevier Inc. All rights reserved.

complete SCI, especially with injuries at C5 or above.

In 2007, Berlly and Shem[3] reported on acute respiratory management after acute SCI. They found that respiratory complications represented 36% of adverse events, and were the most common cause of morbidity in this population. Respiratory failure was the most common cause of mortality in their series, cited in 86% of deaths after acute SCI. Ventilatory failure occurred on average 4.5 days after acute SCI. Hassid and colleagues[4] reviewed nearly 55,000 patients with level I trauma and identified a subgroup of 186 patients with isolated acute cervical SCI. They reported that early intubation for patients with acute complete SCI was mandatory for survival. They favored close observation of patients with incomplete SCI and immediate airway intervention should the patient manifest any evidence of respiratory failure.

BREATHING

Once a definitive airway is achieved it is important to provide ventilatory support to optimize pulmonary function in this patient population. The setting for successful management of cardiovascular and pulmonary support is a dedicated surgical intensive care unit (ICU) where intensivists and surgeons can collaboratively manage patients with SCI. A report spanning a decade of experience with acute traumatic quadriplegia from the National Spinal Injuries Centre in Geneva described 188 patients with acute SCI treated in an ICU setting following immediate transfer from the scene of injury.[5] Through aggressive management in a critical care setting, mortality for complete quadriplegia was reduced from 33% to 7% over the 10-year period. Mortality for patients with incomplete tetraplegia decreased from 10% to less than 2%. Most early deaths in the center's experience were related to pulmonary complications. The likelihood of severe respiratory insufficiency was related to the level and severity of the cervical SCI. Patients with complete injuries had severe respiratory insufficiency in 70% of cases compared with 27% of patients with incomplete lesions. The improvement in mortality rates described was related directly to early monitoring and treatment of respiratory insufficiency in the ICU setting. The investigators stressed that resources for continuous monitoring of central venous pressure, arterial pressure, pulse, respiration rate and pattern, and oxygenation-perfusion parameters were crucial in managing patients with neurologic injuries after acute SCI, particularly those injuries above the C6 level.

Gschaedler and colleagues[6] described the comprehensive management of 51 patients with acute cervical SCIs in an ICU setting in Colmar, France. Forty percent of patients had multiple organ system injuries. They reported a low mortality of 8% and described several severely injured patients who made important neurologic improvements, including 1 Frankel grade A patient who improved to grade D and 2 Frankel grade B patients who changed to grade D. They cited early transport after injury and comprehensive intensive medical care with attention to, and the avoidance of, hypotension and respiratory insufficiency as essential to the improved outcomes their patients experienced. McMichan and colleagues[7] reported a prospective case series of pulmonary complications identified in 22 patients with acute cervical SCI managed in an ICU setting. They compared their results with 22 historical controls with similar injuries. Institution of aggressive pulmonary treatment resulted in zero deaths and fewer respiratory complications compared with those experienced by the retrospective group (9 deaths). They concluded that vigorous pulmonary therapy initiated early after acute SCI was associated with an increased survival rate, a reduced incidence of pulmonary complications, and a decreased need for long ventilatory support.

Pulmonary function has long been known to decline after SCI and especially in those patients with high cervical injuries. This process must be taken into account to change the threshold for intervention because some patients do not meet traditional thresholds for intubation and ventilatory support. One study measured pulmonary function in 16 patients with complete cervical SCI, comparing initial values with those obtained in the same patients at 1, 3, and 5 weeks and 3 and 5 months after injury.[8] In the 1981 report, the investigators noted profound reduction in forced vital capacity (FVC) and expiratory flow rate immediately after injury. Patients with an FVC that was just 25% of expected had a high incidence of respiratory failure requiring ventilator support. This finding was especially true of patients with injuries at C4 or above. FVC was significantly increased at 5 weeks after injury and doubled at 3 months regardless of the level of cervical cord injury. Importantly, hypoxemia (PaO_2 <80 mm Hg) was identified through blood gas analyses in 74% of patients with a low FVC but who did not meet usual criteria for ventilator support determined by normal alveolar ventilation ($PaCO_2$). The investigators attributed this to a ventilation-perfusion imbalance occurring immediately after acute SCI. Systemic hypoxemia responded to treatment with supplemental oxygen in most patients.

Berney and colleagues[9] described their experience with a clinical pathway (classification and decision tree) to direct prolonged intubation and the need for a tracheostomy in 114 patients after acute cervical SCI. The following variables were considered crucial in predicting the need for aggressive airway management: FVC less than 830 mL, need for suction more than every hour, and poor gas exchange (Pao$_2$/fraction of inspired oxygen [Fio$_2$] <188 mm Hg). The use of these variables in the regression analysis allowed accurate prediction of the need for tracheostomy versus successful extubation in 82% of their patients, with fewer than 1 in 10 failing extubation. Overall, a total of 60% of patients required a tracheostomy.

In a subsequent publication, the same group performed a literature review on respiratory complications associated with acute cervical SCI.[10] They identified 21 studies including 1263 patients that described definitive protocols for the respiratory management of acute cervical SCI. Although most of the reports were case series, the investigators discovered that mortality and the risk of respiratory complications were both reduced by 60%, and the need for tracheostomy reduced by 80%, when caregivers/institutions used a respiratory protocol in the management of patients with acute SCI. The use of a clinical pathway reduced the duration of mechanical ventilation by 6 days and ICU length of stay by 7 days.

CIRCULATION

Spinal cord perfusion has long been a topic of interest in patients with SCI. Optimizing perfusion by improving cardiovascular parameters, particularly mean arterial pressure (MAP), is an important step in the care of patients with SCI. Piepmeier and colleagues[11] identified cardiovascular instability after acute cervical SCI in 45 patients they managed in an ICU setting. Twenty-three patients had Frankel grade A injuries, 8 had grade B, 7 had grade C, and 7 had grade D. They discovered a high incidence of cardiovascular irregularities in these patients and identified a direct correlation between the severity of cord injury and incidence and severity of cardiovascular problems. Three patients returned to the ICU setting during the 2-week observation period of the study because of cardiac dysfunction despite a period of initial stability. Twenty-nine of the 45 patients had sustained bradycardia with an average daily pulse rate less than 55 bpm; 32 had episodes during which their pulse rate was less than 50 bpm for a prolonged period of time. Hypotension was common after acute SCI in their series, but most patients responded well to volume replacement. However,

9 patients required vasopressors ranging from a few hours to 5 days to maintain systolic pressure greater than 100 mm Hg. Cardiac arrest occurred in 5 patients (11%). All had Frankel grade A injuries. Three cardiac arrests occurred during respiratory care with endotracheal suctioning. The investigators found that the first week after injury was the time frame during which patients were most vulnerable to cardiovascular instability. Patients with the most severe neurologic injuries were most likely to experience cardiovascular instability after acute SCI regardless of autonomic function. Piepmeier and colleagues[11] concluded that careful monitoring of severely injured patients with acute SCI in the ICU setting reduces the risk of life-threatening emergencies.

Tator and colleagues[12] described their experience with 144 patients with acute SCI managed between 1974 and 1979 at a dedicated SCI unit. They compared their results with a cohort of 358 patients managed between 1948 and 1973 before the development of the acute care SCI facility. All 144 patients managed from 1974 to 1979 were treated in an ICU setting with strict attention to the treatment of hypotension and respiratory failure. Their medical paradigm was developed on the principle that avoiding hypotension is one of the most important aspects of the immediate management of acute cord injury. Hypotension was treated vigorously with crystalloid and transfusion of whole blood or plasma for volume expansion. Patients with respiratory dysfunction were treated with ventilatory support as indicated. Neurologic improvement was observed in 41 of 95 patients (43%) managed under the aggressive ICU medical paradigm. Fifty-two patients (55%) showed no improvement. Only 2 patients (2%) deteriorated. The investigators reported lower mortality, reduced morbidity, shorter length of stay, and lower cost of treatment compared with their earlier experience as a result of this aggressive ICU strategy. They cited improved respiratory management in their ICU as one of the principal factors responsible for reduced mortality and credited the avoidance of hypotension, sepsis, and urologic complications for reduced morbidity after injury.

Lehmann and colleagues[13] reported on a cohort of 71 patients with acute SCI who were managed in an ICU where patients were admitted within 12 hours of SCI and stratified by level and severity of neurologic injury (Frankel scale). Patients were excluded from the cohort if they harbored comorbidities such as head injury, diabetes mellitus, preexisting cardiac disease, or a history of cardiac medication use. The investigators found that all patients with severe cervical SCIs (Frankel grades A and B) had prolonged bradycardia, defined as heart rate less than 60 bpm lasting at least 1 day. Thirty-five percent of Frankel grade C and D patients also showed prolonged bradycardia. Only 13% of patients with thoracic and lumbar SCIs had this finding. In contrast, marked bradycardia (<45 beats per minute [bpm]) was frequent in patients with severe cervical SCI (71%), although less common in patients with more mild cervical (12%) and thoracolumbar (4%) SCI. Sinus node slowing was profound enough to produce hemodynamic compromise and systemic hypotension necessitating bolus injections of atropine or placement of a temporary pacemaker in 29% of the patients with severe cervical SCI. Episodic hypotension unrelated to hypovolemia was identified in 68% of the severe cervical injury group, requiring the use of intravenous pressors in half. Five of 31 patients (16%) in the severe injury group, all with Frankel grade A SCI, experienced a primary cardiac arrest, 3 of which were fatal. There were no significant cardiac rate disturbances or spontaneous episodes of hypotension beyond 14 days of injury. The investigators concluded that potentially life-threatening cardiac arrhythmias and hypotension regularly accompany acute severe injury to the cervical spinal cord within the first 14 days of injury. These events were not solely attributable to disruption of the autonomic nervous system and were best detected and treated in an ICU setting.

Wolf and colleagues[14] described their experience with 52 patients who had bilateral cervical facet dislocation injuries and received ICU care, volume resuscitation, invasive monitoring, and hemodynamic manipulation to maintain MAP greater than 85 mm Hg for 5 days. Thirty-four patients had complete neurologic injuries, 13 had incomplete injuries, and 5 patients were intact neurologically. The investigators attempted closed reduction within 4 hours of patient arrival to their center and performed early open reduction on patients whose injuries could not be reduced by closed means, including closed reduction under anesthesia. All but 3 patients underwent surgery for stabilization and fusion. The investigators reported neurologic improvement at discharge in 21% of the patients with complete SCI and in 62% of patients with incomplete cervical SCI. No intact patient deteriorated. The investigators concluded that their protocol of aggressive, early medical and surgical management of patients with acute SCI improved outcome after injury. Treatment in the ICU setting, hemodynamic monitoring with maintenance of MAP, and early closed or open decompression of the spinal cord were linked to a reduction of secondary complications.

Levi and colleagues[15] treated 50 patients with acute cervical SCI in the ICU according to an aggressive management protocol that included invasive blood pressure monitoring with volume and pharmacologic support to maintain a hemodynamic profile with adequate cardiac output and mean blood pressure of 90 mm Hg. Eight patients had hypotension at the time of admission (systolic blood pressure <90 mm Hg), and 82% of patients developed volume-resistant hypotension that did not respond to volume resuscitation and required pressors within the first 7 days of treatment. This outcome was 5.5 times more common among the patient population that had complete motor injuries. Forty percent of patients managed with increased MAPs, including several with complete injuries, had some degree of neurologic function improvement, 42% remained unchanged, and 18% died. There was minimal morbidity associated with invasive hemodynamic monitoring. The investigators concluded that hemodynamic monitoring in the ICU allows early identification and prompt treatment of cardiac dysfunction and hemodynamic instability and can reduce morbidity and mortality following acute SCI.

Vale and colleagues[16] reported their results from a prospective case series in which aggressive resuscitation and blood pressure management were performed on 77 patients with acute SCI. All patients were managed in the ICU with invasive monitoring (Swan-Ganz catheters and arterial lines) and blood pressure augmentation to maintain MAP greater than 85 mm Hg for 7 days after injury. They reported 10 patients with complete cervical SCI (American Spinal Injury Association [ASIA] grade A), 25 with incomplete cervical injuries (ASIA grades B, C, and D), 21 patients with complete thoracic SCI, and 8 patients with incomplete thoracic-level SCI (grades B, C, and D). The average admission MAP for ASIA A cervical patients was 66 mm Hg; 90% of these patients required pressors in addition to volume replacement to maintain an MAP of 85 mm Hg or greater. Fifty-two percent of patients with incomplete cervical SCI required pressors to maintain MAP at 85 mm Hg. Only 9 of 29 patients with thoracic-level SCI required the use of pressors. The investigators reported minimal morbidity with the use of invasive monitoring or with pharmacologic therapy to augment MAP. At 1-year follow-up (mean, 17 months), neurologic recovery was variable and typically incomplete. Three of 10 cervical ASIA A patients regained ambulatory capacity, and 2 regained bladder function. Twenty-three of the patients with incomplete cervical SCI regained ambulatory function at 12 months of follow-up, only 4 of whom had initial examination scores consistent with the ability to ambulate. Twenty-two of 25 patients (88%) regained bladder control. Thirty-one of 35 patients with cervical SCI and 27 of 29 with thoracic-level injury were treated surgically. The investigators compared surgical treatment, early and late, with neurologic outcome and found no statistical correlation. They concluded that the enhanced neurologic outcome identified in their series after acute SCI was optimized by early and aggressive volume resuscitation and blood pressure augmentation and was in addition to and/or distinct from any potential benefit provided by surgery.

Guly and colleagues[17] found an incidence of systolic blood pressure less than 100 mm Hg and heart rate less than 80 bpm (ie, neurologic shock) of 19.3% (95% confidence interval, 14.8–23.7) in a series of 490 patients with acute SCI. In 2006, Franga and colleagues[18] described an incidence of cardiovascular instability of 17%, including bradyarrhythmias requiring permanent pacemaker placement, among 30 patients with acute complete cervical SCI.

SUMMARY OF THE ABCs

Patients with acute SCI, particularly cervical injuries, frequently develop hypotension, hypoxemia, pulmonary dysfunction, and cardiovascular instability, often despite initially stable cardiac and pulmonary function. These complications are not limited to patients with complete SCI. Life-threatening cardiovascular instability and respiratory insufficiency may be transient and episodic and may be recurrent in the first 7 to 10 days after injury. Patients with the most severe neurologic injuries seem to have the greatest risk of these life-threatening events. Evidence indicates that ICU monitoring allows the early detection of hemodynamic instability, cardiac disturbances, pulmonary dysfunction, and hypoxemia. Prompt treatment of these events in patients with acute SCI reduces cardiac-related and respiratory-related morbidity and mortality.

Management in an ICU or other monitored setting seems to have a positive impact on neurologic outcome after acute cervical SCI. Invasive arterial monitoring may also have a role in improving neurologic function. Retrospective studies consistently report that volume expansion and blood pressure augmentation performed under controlled circumstances in an ICU setting are linked to improved ASIA scores in patients with acute SCI compared with historical controls. Evidence suggests that the maintenance of MAP at 85 to 90 mm Hg after acute SCI for a duration

of 7 days is safe and may improve spinal cord perfusion and ultimately neurologic outcome.

CLOSED REDUCTION

Once the ABCs have been addressed, restoration of normal anatomic alignment (decompression) is the next goal in patients with SCI. The 2002 report from the Joint Section on Disorders of the Spine and Peripheral Nerves of the American Association of Neurological Surgeons/Congress of Neurological Surgeons published an evidence-based guideline on the issue of closed reduction.[19] That review reported the efficacy of closed reduction of acute cervical spinal fracture-dislocation injuries derived from combined case series published in the literature: 1200 patients were treated with closed reduction, 80% successfully. The reported rate of permanent neurologic deterioration was less than 1% and the rate of transient injury was between 2% and 4%. Although there was insufficient evidence to support a standard of care or establish a clinical guideline, the investigators concluded that "early closed reduction of cervical spine fracture-dislocation injuries with craniocervical traction is recommended to restore anatomic alignment of the cervical spine in awake patients."[19]

Several additional case series were subsequently published and were added to the updated guidelines in 2013, involving an additional 195 patients.[20] Beyer and colleagues[21] described their experience with 34 patients, 28 of whom were treated with attempted closed reduction. Only 10 of 28 injuries were completely reduced with halo traction and achieved anatomic realignment; 7 injuries could not be reduced at all. The investigators described greater difficulty with the reduction of unilateral facet dislocation injuries. O'Connor and colleagues[22] reported 21 patients with subaxial cervical facet injuries treated with attempted closed reduction; 11 patients had successful reduction of their injuries. Closed reduction was not successful in fracture-dislocation injuries more than 5 days old (n = 5). One patient experienced transient neurologic deterioration. Koivikko and colleagues[23] successfully reduced cervical fracture-dislocation injuries in 62 of 85 patients (73%) they treated with craniocervical traction; 1 of those experienced neurologic deterioration during successful reduction.

In another retrospective series of 45 patients undergoing closed reduction of unilateral and bilateral traumatic cervical spinal facet dislocation injuries, 89% were successful.[24] Time to reduction did not correlate with improved motor score outcome. Reindl and colleagues[25] reported 80% success in 41 patients treated with closed reduction before surgery. One patient had transient neurologic deterioration caused by closed reduction that had resolved at 1 year after surgery. Evidence generally supports the efficacy of closed reduction of acute traumatic cervical spinal fracture-dislocation injuries, but a definitive improvement in neurologic outcome has yet to be proved by randomized controlled trials.

Hence, in 2013, the guidelines committee again concluded that closed reduction of fracture-dislocation injuries of the cervical spine by traction-reduction seems to be safe and effective for the reduction of acute traumatic spinal deformity in awake patients.[19] A review of the literature suggests that up to 80% of patients have their cervical fracture-dislocation injuries reduced with this technique, with an overall permanent neurologic complication rate of closed reduction of 1%. However, reduction must be carefully performed in a supervised setting on awake and cooperative patients by specialists trained in the techniques of reduction.

Case Example

A 68-year-old woman fell from a horse, incurring a flexion-distraction injury with a left-sided unilateral jumped facet at C5-C6 (**Fig. 1**). Neurologic examination revealed a capelike pattern of dysesthesia and diffuse 4/5 strength in the upper extremities but normal sensory and motor examinations in the lower extremities. She was placed in Gardner-Wells tongs and sequential weights were added until she was in 23 kg (50 lb) of in-line traction; we completed a neurologic examination between each addition of weight. Using lateral fluoroscopy and manual manipulation, we successfully reduced the left C5-C6 facet (**Fig. 2**). The patient's neurologic examination remained stable throughout this procedure. In the operating room, she underwent C5-C6 anterior cervical discectomy and interbody placement. Given the disruption of her facets bilaterally, she then underwent a C5-C6 posterior spinal instrumentation and arthrodesis (**Fig. 3**). Postoperatively, her MAPs were kept greater than 85 mm Hg for 3 days and her symptoms gradually improved to near full strength.

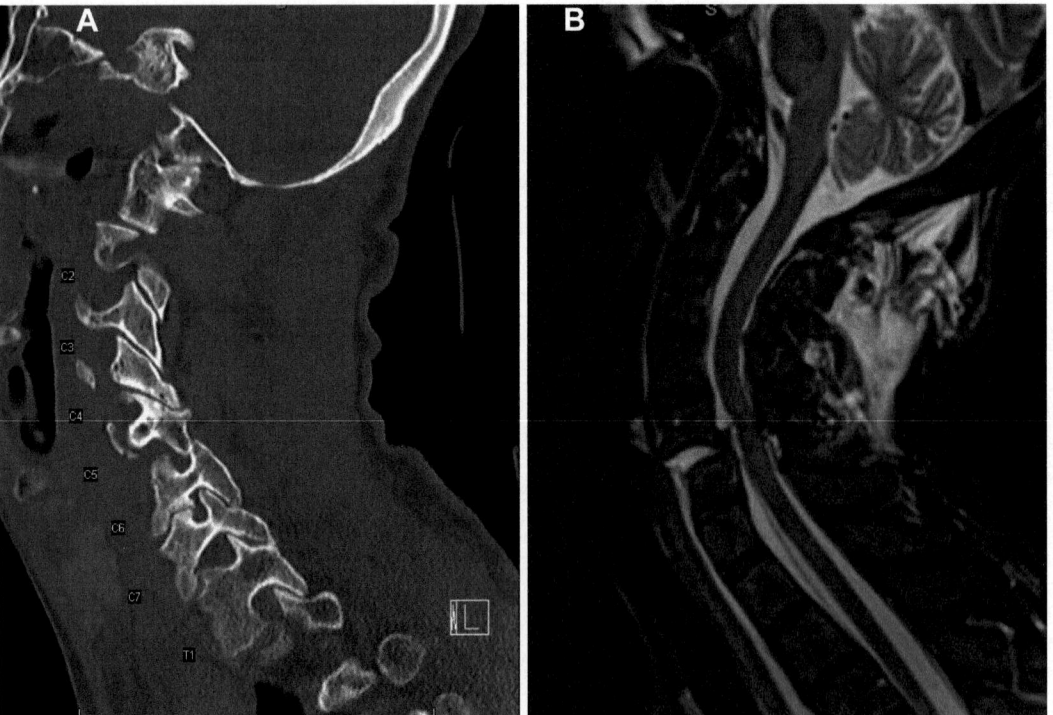

Fig. 1. (*A*) Sagittal paramedian computed tomography showing the left C5-C6 facet in jumped and locked configuration. (*B*) Sagittal T2-weighted midline MRI showing disruption of the C5-C6 intervertebral disc without significant herniation into the canal, disruption of the anterior and posterior longitudinal ligaments, and T2 signal showing soft tissue edema of the paraspinal musculature.

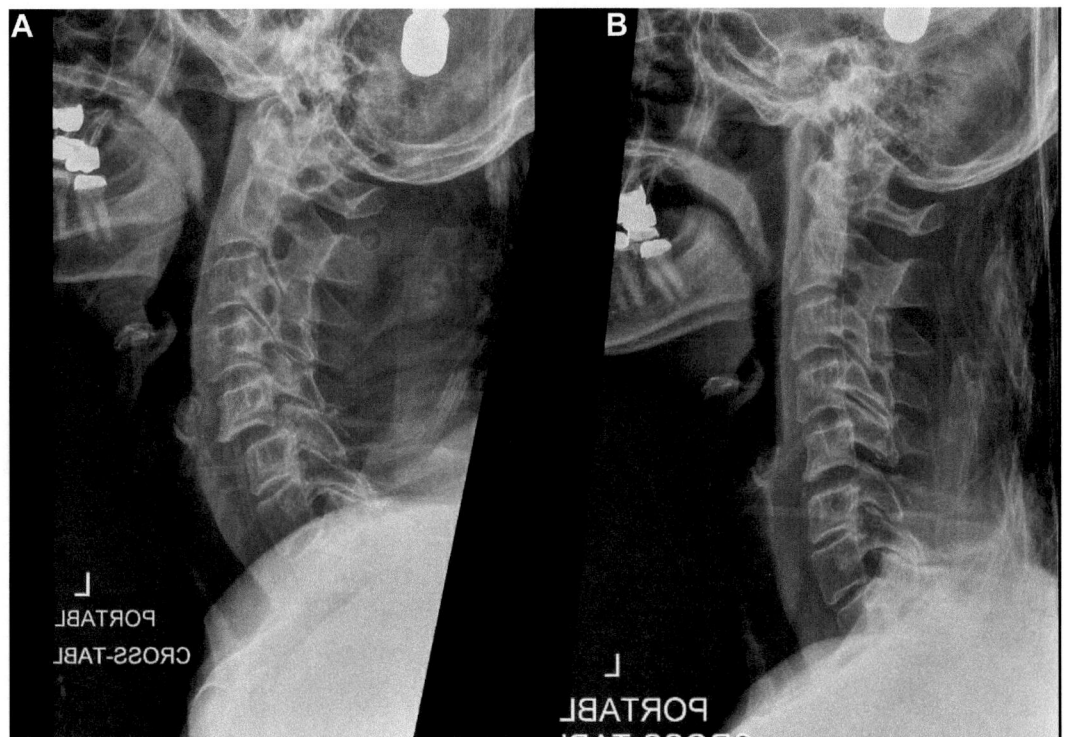

Fig. 2. (*A*) Prereduction lateral fluoroscopic image showing anterolisthesis of C5 on C6. (*B*) Postreduction lateral fluoroscopic image with the patient in 23 kg (50 lb) of in-line traction showing closed reduction of the injury with restoration of spinal alignment.

PREREDUCTION MRI

The role of MRI before closed or open posterior reduction remains controversial. There are isolated reports in the literature of deterioration of neurologic function during or immediately after these maneuvers. This finding has led some clinicians to recommend universal MRI screening of all patients before reduction, looking for canal stenosis from herniated disk fragments. However, there are several drawbacks to this algorithm as well. Delay in definitive cord decompression can occur if there are delays caused by scheduling and image acquisition. In addition, the transfer of patients with unstable spine injuries from bed into the MR scanner creates additional risk.

The clinical importance of MRI-documented disk herniation or protrusion in association with cervical facet injury is unknown. A series of 37 patients managed with closed reduction showed a disk herniation in 9 patients, 4 of whom underwent later anterior decompression.[26] A subsequent series of 13 patients drawn from 4 institutions over an unspecified time period in which every patient had an MRI study at some point during their care showed 10 patients with herniated discs and 3 with bulging discs at the level of injury,[27] calling

into question the clinical significance of this finding. None of the patients in the study developed a new permanent neurologic deficit during or after closed reduction maneuvers. One study in the literature specifically involved the use of prereduction and postreduction MRI; the investigators found that 3 of 9 patients had new disc herniations after closed reduction, but none of those patients deteriorated neurologically.[28] In a larger series of 80 patients in whom MRI scans were acquired after closed reduction, 46% had herniated or bulging discs, but only 1 patient had temporary worsening of a radiculopathy after closed reduction.[29] In addition, a series by Rizzolo and colleagues[30] showed that 55% of patients with cervical SCI had a disc disruption or herniation. Patients in this series who were awake and able to report neurologic changes during closed reduction underwent the maneuver; none of them had further loss of neurologic function. Patients who were not awake or alert enough to reliably participate in an examination did not undergo closed reduction. All of these studies call into question the clinical significance of MRI findings in guiding management.

In 2006, Darsaut and colleagues[31] reported experience with a unique traction device that

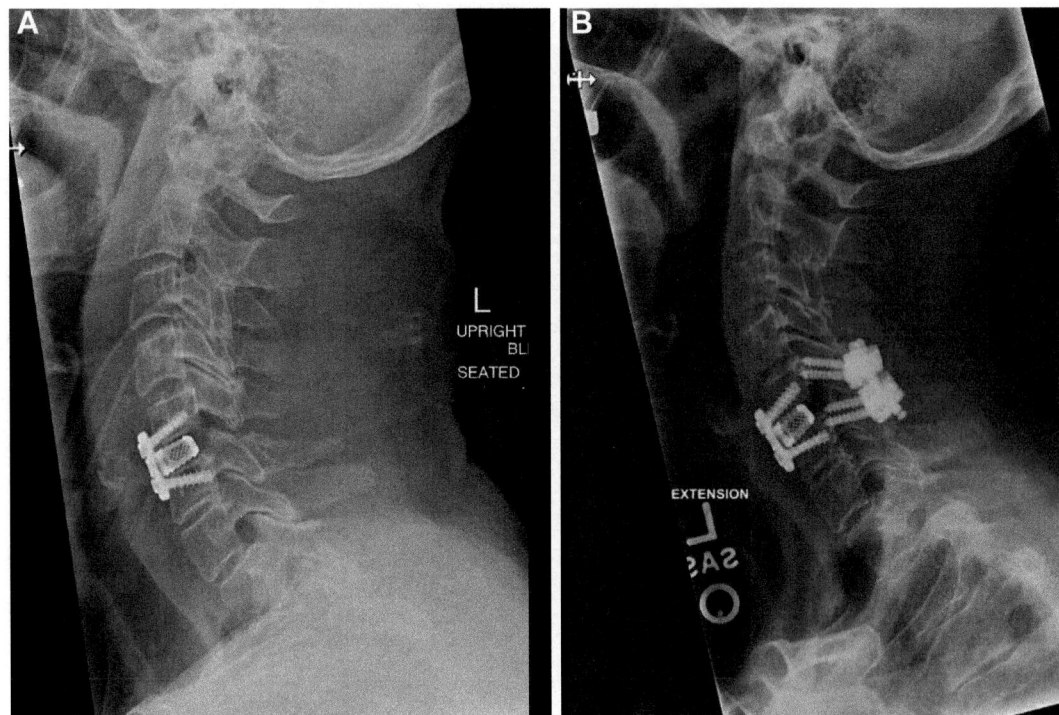

Fig. 3. (*A*) Upright cervical spine lateral plain film showing postoperative changes from C5-C6 anterior cervical discectomy and interbody placement with widening of C5-C6 facets. (*B*) Upright cervical spine lateral plain film showing postoperative changes from C5-C6 posterior spinal instrumentation and arthrodesis showing compression between C5-C6 facets.

allowed monitoring of closed reduction using MRI. Seventeen nonconsecutive patients were studied; 11 of 17 injuries were successfully reduced with closed traction. Nine of those 11 patients achieved simultaneous complete spinal cord decompression. One patient had incomplete decompression, and 1 patient had persisting cord compression despite realignment. All soft disk herniations identified before the initiation of closed reduction were reduced back into the disk space as part of the traction-reduction process.

Despite the paucity of evidence regarding the value of prereduction MRI in patients with cervical spinal dislocation, the topic remains controversial. Lee and colleagues[32] in 2009 published a review on the topic and found no medical evidence-based guidelines for the treatment of obtunded patients with a cervical dislocation. Arnold and colleagues[33] performed a survey of 29 spinal surgeons from The Spine Trauma Study Group asking for their management responses to 10 clinical scenarios related to acute unilateral and bilateral cervical facet dislocation injuries. There was substantial variability among surgeons regarding the need for prereduction MRI, depending on the clinical scenario (42%–77%), and little agreement regarding open or closed reduction to reduce the

injury or the operative approach to provide definitive surgical treatment. In 2004, Koivikko and colleagues[23] reported their experiences with a series of 85 patients treated for cervical fracture-dislocation injuries. Sixty-two experienced successful reduction with closed cervical traction; the others required operative reduction. No patients underwent prereduction MRI, and no patient deteriorated neurologically as a result of closed reduction. All surgical patients were treated with posterior interspinous wiring with fusion. Despite these results, the investigators admit to more recent use of prereduction MRI in the management of patients with cervical fracture-dislocations since their publication.

Neurologic deterioration from extruded disk material has been reported to occur in conjunction with both anterior and posterior open reduction following failed closed reduction. Eismont and colleagues[34] reported a series of 63 patients managed with closed traction-reduction followed by open reduction if closed reduction was unsuccessful. One of these patients worsened following posterior open reduction and fusion. A herniated disk was found ventral to the cord on postprocedure myelography. Herniated disks were found in 3 other patients who failed closed reduction and in 2 patients with static neurologic deficits following fracture-dislocation reduction (1 open, 1 closed). One of these patients deteriorated after subsequent anterior cervical diskectomy and fusion. In another report, 2 patients were found to have disk herniations on postreduction imaging, with both patients deteriorating after open reduction following failure of attempted closed reduction.[35] Robertson and Ryan[36] reported 3 patients who deteriorated during management of cervical subluxation injuries and 1 that deteriorated en route to the medical center and was found to have a disk herniation in the canal causing severe stenosis. The second of the 3, who had a loss of neurologic function after open posterior reduction and instrumentation/arthrodesis, was also shown to have herniated disc fragments causing spinal cord compression. The third had deterioration after a closed reduction technique with a disc herniation revealed on the postreduction MRI. One more substantial review of 16 patients that had neurologic compromise after closed or open posterior reduction of facet dislocations attempted to describe the spectrum of the severity of deterioration. Seven of the 16 patients developed complete cord injuries. Six of these were after open posterior reduction and 1 followed manipulation under anesthesia.[37] There are only 2 documented cases of neurologic deterioration associated with attempted closed reduction of cervical spine fracture-dislocation injuries resulting from cord compression from disk herniation.[38,39]

Prereduction MRI shows disc herniations in up to half of all patients with cervical spine facet subluxation, but the clinical significance is unclear. There is a general lack of correlation between the presence of herniated disc material and the likelihood of neurologic deterioration after closed reduction or open posterior reduction techniques. Given the lack of evidence supporting its use, the potential benefit must be weighed against the risks of delaying definitive treatment of the injury and risks of the transportation of unstable spinal injuries. The American Association of Neurological Surgeons Guidelines on Management of Spinal Cord Injury states that there is class III medical evidence that supports early closed reduction of cervical fracture-dislocation injuries with respect to neurologic recovery and do not specifically recommend obtaining a prereduction MRI. One patient population in which prereduction MRI might be beneficial is that with obtunded SCI requiring restoration of normal anatomic spinal alignment. The other indication for prereduction MRI is an open reduction of an unreducible injury, particularly if a posterior approach is needed for successful reduction.

TIMING OF SURGICAL MANAGEMENT

Evidence in the literature increasingly supports early surgical intervention after traumatic SCI. The largest high-quality study to date examining this question, the Surgical Timing in Acute Spinal Cord Injury Study (STASCIS), defined early surgery as less than 24 hours after the initial injury.[40] The investigators found that, after adjusting for variables such as preoperative neurologic status or administration of steroids, patients who underwent early surgical decompression and arthrodesis had a 2.8 times higher likelihood of having at least a 2-grade improvement in ASIA Impairment Scale score. Although this was a prospective but nonrandomized study, a compelling argument was made for early surgical intervention. Patients who underwent early surgery were more likely to have an initial motor assessment of complete injury, suggesting that even patients with these injuries could have benefit (ASIA A or B vs C, D, or E; 58% vs 38%). Timing for truly complete injuries (ASIA A) remains controversial. An observational cohort study specifically examining timing of surgery (<24 hours vs >24 hours) and motor recovery in complete cervical injuries did not show any benefit to patients with this metric whether patients underwent early surgical intervention or not.[41] This finding has been supported by several other studies in populations with thoracic and cervical injuries.[42]

SUMMARY

Immediate attention to the ABCs in the field and in the hospital forms the cornerstone of managing acute SCI. ICU care involving oxygenation, airway and ventilation support, and hemodynamic augmentation is repeatedly reported to improve survival, reduce complications, and improve neurologic outcomes. Early reduction and decompression of the compressed spinal cord by closed or open means provides the best opportunity for improvement in the setting of incomplete SCI.

CLINICS CARE POINTS

- Patients with cervical cord injury have high rates of respiratory failure and require close monitoring in an ICU. Up to 60% require intubation and/or tracheostomy.
- Life-threatening arrythmias and hypotension accompany severe cervical SCI.

- Early closed reduction of cervical spine fracture dislocation injuries can be performed safely with up to 80% of patients achieving successful reduction.

- The role of prereduction MRI remains controversial, with up to 50% of patients who achieve successful and safe closed reduction demonstrating a prereduction disc herniation.

- The use of prereduction MRI should be strongly considered in obtunded patients or those who have had unsuccessful attempts at closed reduction prior to proceeding to surgical reduction.

DISCLOSURE

The authors have nothing to disclose.

REFERENCES

1. Jain NB, Ayers GD, Peterson EN, et al. Traumatic spinal cord injury in the United States, 1993-2012. JAMA 2015;313(22):2236–43.
2. Como JJ, Sutton ER, McCunn M, et al. Characterizing the need for mechanical ventilation following cervical spinal cord injury with neurologic deficit. J Trauma 2005;59(4):912–6 [discussion: 916].
3. Berlly M, Shem K. Respiratory management during the first five days after spinal cord injury. J Spinal Cord Med 2007;30(4):309–18.
4. Hassid VJ, Schinco MA, Tepas JJ, et al. Definitive establishment of airway control is critical for optimal outcome in lower cervical spinal cord injury. J Trauma 2008;65(6):1328–32.
5. Hachen HJ. Idealized care of the acutely injured spinal cord in Switzerland. J Trauma 1977;17(12): 931–6.
6. Gschaedler R, Dollfus P, Mole JP, et al. Reflections on the intensive care of acute cervical spinal cord injuries in a general traumatology centre. Paraplegia 1979;17(1):58–61.
7. McMichan JC, Michel L, Westbrook PR. Pulmonary dysfunction following traumatic quadriplegia. Recognition, prevention, and treatment. JAMA 1980;243(6):528–31.
8. Ledsome JR, Sharp JM. Pulmonary function in acute cervical cord injury. Am Rev Respir Dis 1981;124(1): 41–4.
9. Berney SC, Gordon IR, Opdam HI, et al. A classification and regression tree to assist clinical decision making in airway management for patients with cervical spinal cord injury. Spinal Cord 2011; 49(2):244–50.
10. Berney S, Bragge P, Granger C, et al. The acute respiratory management of cervical spinal cord injury in the first 6 weeks after injury: a systematic review. Spinal Cord 2011;49(1):17–29.
11. Piepmeier JM, Lehmann KB, Lane JG. Cardiovascular instability following acute cervical spinal cord trauma. Cent Nerv Syst Trauma 1985;2(3):153–60.
12. Tator CH, Rowed DW, Schwartz ML, et al. Management of acute spinal cord injuries. Can J Surg 1984;27(3):289–93, 296.
13. Lehmann KG, Lane JG, Piepmeier JM, et al. Cardiovascular abnormalities accompanying acute spinal cord injury in humans: incidence, time course and severity. J Am Coll Cardiol 1987;10(1):46–52.
14. Wolf A, Levi L, Mirvis S, et al. Operative management of bilateral facet dislocation. J Neurosurg 1991;75(6):883–90.
15. Levi L, Wolf A, Belzberg H. Hemodynamic parameters in patients with acute cervical cord trauma: description, intervention, and prediction of outcome. Neurosurgery 1993;33(6):1007–16 [discussion: 1016–7].
16. Vale FL, Burns J, Jackson AB, et al. Combined medical and surgical treatment after acute spinal cord injury: results of a prospective pilot study to assess the merits of aggressive medical resuscitation and blood pressure management. J Neurosurg 1997; 87(2):239–46.
17. Guly HR, Bouamra O, Lecky FE, et al. The incidence of neurogenic shock in patients with isolated spinal cord injury in the emergency department. Resuscitation 2008;76(1):57–62.
18. Franga DL, Hawkins ML, Medeiros RS, et al. Recurrent asystole resulting from high cervical spinal cord injuries. Am Surg 2006;72(6):525–9.
19. Hadley MN, Walters BC, Grabb BC, et al. Initial closed reduction of cervical spine fracture-dislocation injuries. Neurosurgery 2002;50(3 Suppl):S44–50.
20. Gelb DE, Hadley MN, Aarabi B, et al. Initial closed reduction of cervical spinal fracture-dislocation injuries. Neurosurgery 2013;72(Suppl 2):73–83.
21. Beyer CA, Cabanela ME. Unilateral facet dislocations and fracture-dislocations of the cervical spine: a review. Orthopedics 1992;15(3):311–5.
22. O'Connor PA, McCormack O, Noel J, et al. Anterior displacement correlates with neurological impairment in cervical facet dislocations. Int Orthop 2003;27(3):190–3.
23. Koivikko MP, Myllynen P, Santavirta S. Fracture dislocations of the cervical spine: a review of 106 conservatively and operatively treated patients. Eur Spine J 2004;13(7):610–6.
24. Greg Anderson D, Voets C, Ropiak R, et al. Analysis of patient variables affecting neurologic outcome after traumatic cervical facet dislocation. Spine J 2004;4(5):506–12.

25. Reindl R, Ouellet J, Harvey EJ, et al. Anterior reduction for cervical spine dislocation. Spine (Phila Pa 1976) 2006;31(6):648–52.

26. Harrington JF, Likavec MJ, Smith AS. Disc herniation in cervical fracture subluxation. Neurosurgery 1991; 29(3):374–9.

27. Doran SE, Papadopoulos SM, Ducker TB, et al. Magnetic resonance imaging documentation of coexistent traumatic locked facets of the cervical spine and disc herniation. J Neurosurg 1993;79(3):341–5.

28. Vaccaro AR, Falatyn SP, Flanders AE. Magnetic resonance evaluation of the intervertebral disc, spinal ligaments, and spinal cord before and after closed traction reduction of cervical spine dislocations. Spine (Phila Pa 1976) 1999;24(12):1210–7.

29. Grant GA, Mirza SK, Chapman JR, et al. Risk of early closed reduction in cervical spine subluxation injuries. J Neurosurg 1999;90(1 Suppl):13–8.

30. Rizzolo SJ, Vaccaro AR, Cotler JM. Cervical spine trauma. Spine (Phila Pa 1976) 1994;19(20):2288–98.

31. Darsaut TE, Ashforth R, Bhargava R, et al. A pilot study of magnetic resonance imaging-guided closed reduction of cervical spine fractures. Spine (Phila Pa 1976) 2006;31(18):2085–90.

32. Lee JY, Nassr A, Eck JC, et al. Controversies in the treatment of cervical spine dislocations. Spine J 2009;9(5):418–23.

33. Arnold PM, Brodke DS, Rampersaud YR, et al. Differences between neurosurgeons and orthopedic surgeons in classifying cervical dislocation injuries and making assessment and treatment decisions: a multicenter reliability study. Am J Orthop (Belle Mead NJ) 2009;38(10):E156–61.

34. Eismont FJ, Arena MJ, Green BA. Extrusion of an intervertebral disc associated with traumatic subluxation or dislocation of cervical facets. Case report. J Bone Joint Surg Am 1991;73(10):1555–60.

35. Olerud C, Jonsson H Jr. Compression of the cervical spine cord after reduction of fracture dislocations. Report of 2 cases. Acta Orthop Scand 1991;62(6): 599–601.

36. Robertson PA, Ryan MD. Neurological deterioration after reduction of cervical subluxation. Mechanical compression by disc tissue. J Bone Joint Surg Br 1992;74(2):224–7.

37. Mahale YJ, Silver JR, Henderson NJ. Neurological complications of the reduction of cervical spine dislocations. J Bone Joint Surg Br 1993;75(3): 403–9.

38. Maiman DJ, Barolat G, Larson SJ. Management of bilateral locked facets of the cervical spine. Neurosurgery 1986;18(5):542–7.

39. Farmer J, Vaccaro A, Albert TJ, et al. Neurologic deterioration after cervical spinal cord injury. J Spinal Disord 1998;11(3):192–6.

40. Fehlings MG, Vaccaro A, Wilson JR, et al. Early versus delayed decompression for traumatic cervical spinal cord injury: results of the Surgical Timing in Acute Spinal Cord Injury Study (STASCIS). PLoS One 2012;7(2):e32037.

41. Dvorak MF, Noonan VK, Fallah N, et al. The influence of time from injury to surgery on motor recovery and length of hospital stay in acute traumatic spinal cord injury: an observational Canadian cohort study. J Neurotrauma 2015;32(9):645–54.

42. Petitjean ME, Mousselard H, Pointillart V, et al. Thoracic spinal trauma and associated injuries: should early spinal decompression be considered? J Trauma 1995;39(2):368–72.

Central Cord Syndrome Redefined

Mauricio J. Avila, MD, R. John Hurlbert, MD, PhD*

KEYWORDS

- Central cord syndrome • Cervical spondylosis • Cervical stenosis • Spinal cord injury • Elderly
- Falls • Neck trauma • Hyperextension

KEY POINTS

- Difficulties defining central cord syndrome based on neurologic examination interfere with obtaining accurate population-based demographic and outcome data.
- Central cord syndrome is characterized by low-velocity/low-impact trauma in the setting of preexisting spondylosis resulting in spinal cord injury without fracture or dislocation.
- The pathophysiology of central cord syndrome likely involves transverse shear forces originating in the central gray matter, spreading lateral toward descending white matter tracts proportional to injury intensity.
- Central cord syndrome involves a spectrum of neurologic deficits preferentially affecting the hands and arms, but ranging from mild paresthesias in the hands to complete quadriplegia in its most severe form.

INTRODUCTION

Spinal cord injury (SCI) encompasses a broad spectrum of neurologic deficits resulting from trauma to the spinal column. Several syndromes associated with SCI have been identified to indicate unique neurologic deficits arising from injury to specific tracts within the spinal cord. Anterior cord syndrome is associated with occlusion of the anterior spinal artery and typically involves a dense motor deficit, absent light touch and pain appreciation, but preservation of dorsal column deep pressure and position sensation.[1] In contrast a posterior cord syndrome can result from occlusion of the posterior spinal arteries and is characterized by dorsal column deficits (ataxia) but preserved motor, light touch, and pain function. Brown-Séquard syndrome can occur from penetrating trauma and denotes lateral SCI resulting in ipsilateral motor and dorsal column deficits, and contralateral light touch and pain deficits.[2] Conus medullaris syndrome arises from trauma to the conus in the region of L1 or L2, resulting in various degrees of paraplegia including sensory and sphincter impairment, but with lower motor neuron characteristics including hypotonia, hyporeflexia, and urinary retention.[1] Of the different SCI patterns, central cord syndrome (CCS) represents the most common form of incomplete SCI.[3]

The first description of a patient with CCS was published by Sir William Thorburn, a general surgeon at the Manchester Royal Infirmary in Manchester, England (**Fig. 1**A). In the preradiograph era of the late 1800s he reported a series of nine cervical spinal cord injuries in which one patient demonstrated hand function to be more severely affected than leg function.[4] Thorburn postulated this unique injury pattern to arise from hemorrhage into the central gray matter of the spinal cord, but because the patient survived was unable to confirm his suspicions on necropsy.

It was not until more than 60 years later that Richard Schneider (**Fig. 1**B), a neurosurgeon at the University of Michigan, identified Thorburn's original case and reported a series of additional

Department of Neurosurgery, University of Arizona, Banner University Medical Center, PO Box 245070, 1501 North Campbell Avenue, Room 4303, Tucson, AZ 85724-5070, USA
* Corresponding author.
E-mail address: rjhurlbert@neurosurgery.arizona.edu

Neurosurg Clin N Am 32 (2021) 353–363
https://doi.org/10.1016/j.nec.2021.03.007

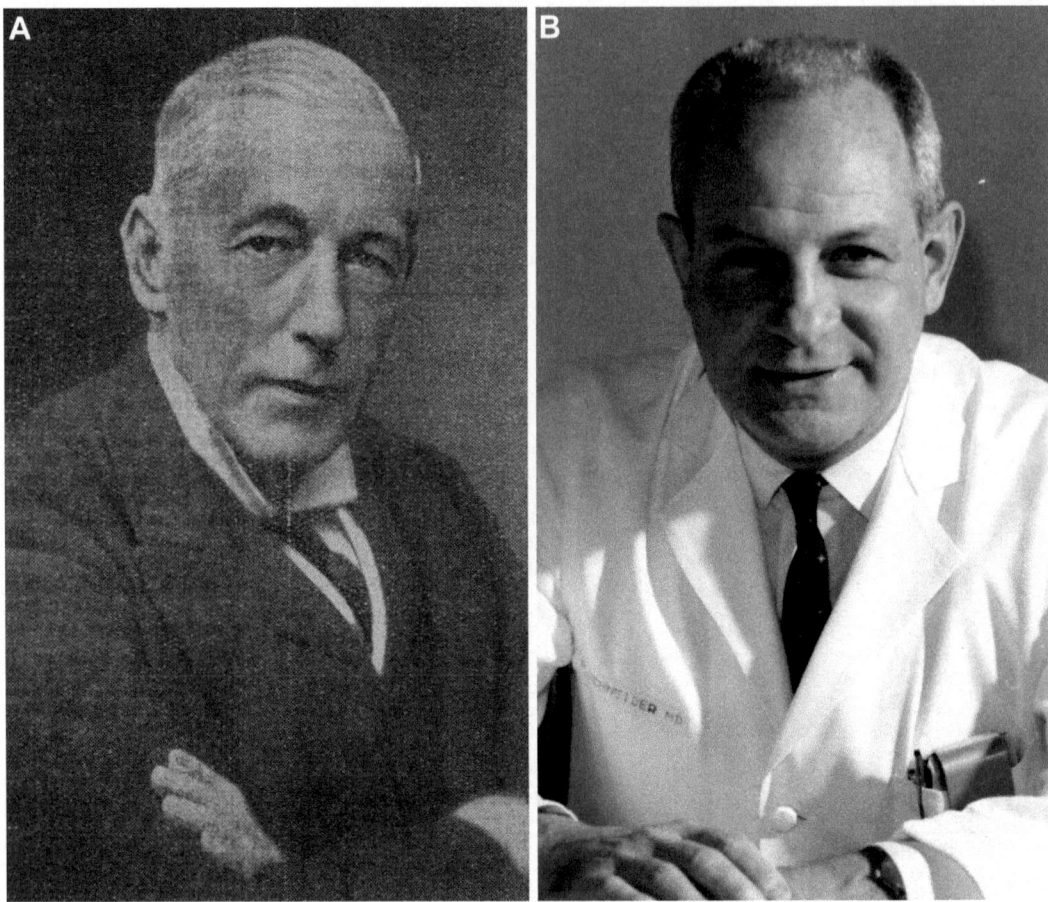

Fig. 1. (*A*) Sir William Thorburn (1861–1923), a general surgeon working at the Manchester Royal Infirmary with a special interest in spinal injuries, provided the first case report of a patient with post-traumatic paralysis 178 involving the hands more than the legs in 1887. (*B*) Dr Richard Schneider (1913–1986), a neurosurgeon in Ann Arbor at the University of Michigan, defined and characterized "central cord syndrome" as a unique form of incomplete spinal cord injury. (*From* [A] THE LATE SIR WILLIAM THORBURN. *Br Med J.* 1923;1(3248):576-577; and [B] From Bentley Historical Library, University of Michigan; with permission.)

patients with cervical SCI similarly affected by hand greater than arm or leg dysfunction, introducing the term "syndrome of acute central cervical cord injury."[5] He identified this syndrome as characterized by "disproportionately more motor impairment of the upper than of the lower extremities, bladder dysfunction, usually urinary retention, and varying degrees of sensory loss below the level of the lesion."[5] He was also able to conclude that the injury typically involved an extension mechanism.

Almost 70 years since Schneider's original description, the definition of CCS has remained largely unaltered: an acute cervical SCI disproportionately affecting the hands compared with the more proximal upper and the lower extremities. Today the diagnosis of CCS remains anchored to the neurologic examination.[3] However, this has

led to considerable confusion in reliably diagnosing CCS, which naturally involves a spectrum of injury severities. Some patients present with only tingling in their hands and fingers but are otherwise neurologically intact and never admitted to hospital. Others present with near-quadriplegia demonstrating profound residual hand and leg paralysis even after months of rehabilitation and recovery. Hence epidemiologic and outcome information for patients with CSS is largely missing; available data are contaminated by patients with generic SCI caused by more traditional fracture dislocations. In a new era of "big data" with an aging population and CSS on the rise, it is more important than ever to distinguish this mechanism of SCI from others so that it is diagnosed, studied, and treated appropriately for the unique syndrome it represents.

In this review we revisit the epidemiologic factors that relate to CCS, explore the pathophysiology behind it, and compare outcomes with more traditional SCI. We conclude by proposing a modernized definition of CCS hoping to set the stage for ease of diagnosis in a homogenous population, ultimately permitting better research and consistency in management strategies.

EPIDEMIOLOGY

Bosch and colleagues[6] estimated the incidence of CCS to be approximately 10% of all traumatic cord injuries and 20% of cervical injuries in their series of 447 patients with SCI admitted to Ranchos Los Amigos hospital between 1955 and 1965. Four decades later McKinley and colleagues[7] identified 44% of 839 consecutive patients with SCI admitted for rehabilitation at Virginia Commonwealth University between 1992 and 2004 as having CCS. Patients with CCS were older compared with the other SCI syndromes. The mechanism of injury in CSS was commonly low-speed/low-impact trauma (eg, ground level fall) compared with high-impact trauma causing fracture dislocations. McKinley and colleagues[7] also observed the most common level of neurologic injury sustained in CSS to be C4 and C5. Other studies have confirmed CCS to occur without fracture or dislocation as a result of an extension injury from low-impact trauma in an older population with preexisting cervical stenosis.[8–10]

From a broader perspective, larger databases show demographic characteristics of all SCI to be in evolution over the past several decades. Hagen and coworkers[11] reported an increase in the incidence of SCI in Norway, quadrupling from 6.2 cases per million population in the 1950s to 26.2 cases per million in 2001. During the same time period the mean age of those injured rose from 40 to 49 years.[11] Of note, is that patients 50 years and older were more likely to suffer an incomplete injury of the cervical spine. Ahoniemi and colleagues[12] undertook a similar study in Finland, reporting a parallel increase in the incidence of SCI from 13 to 24 cases per million over 30 years between 1970 and 2000. During this time period the mean age of Finnish patients with SCI rose from 37 to 42 years, whereas the incidence of SCI in people 55 and older doubled.[12] Comparing cohorts from 1995 to 1998 with 2009 to 2013, Toda and colleagues[13] found the incidence of SCI in patients 60 and older to also have doubled in Japan. Similar to the trends reported in Norway, they noted these older patients

to more frequently suffer cervical injuries of an incomplete nature.

The United States typically reports the highest incidence of SCI compared with other countries, recently estimated to be 17,000 new cases per year (54 cases per million population).[14–16] The demographics of SCI in this country are similarly evolving toward a predominantly older population.[14,17] Data from the National Spinal Cord Injury Statistical Center shows that mean age for SCI has shifted from 29 years of age in the 1970s to 43 years in 2018.[16]

In summary, diverse populations throughout the world confirm the rising incidence of SCI because of more injuries in older people from less violent trauma. These injuries more frequently involve the cervical spine and more often result in an incomplete neurologic deficit. It is possible that in the twenty-first century, CCS accounts for more than half of all SCI. Difficulties with accurate diagnosis and reliable reporting currently prevent the granularity necessary to identify CSS on a national scale.

PATHOPHYSIOLOGY

A major barrier to better understanding the pathophysiology and natural history of CCS arises from inconsistencies within patient populations reported in the literature. Beginning with Schneider's original series in the 1950s and continuing through today,[18] reports of CCS encompass a mix of patients with cervical spondylosis, Ossification of the Posterior Longitudinal Ligament (OPLL), traumatic disk herniations, and patients with fracture/subluxations.[5]

Schneider's original description proposed the mechanism of CCS to be a hyperextension injury causing spinal cord compression between anterior osteophytes and posterior ligamentum flavum, with or without actual fracture to the spine.[5] Lending evidence to this theory is a study by Taylor[19] published a few years earlier demonstrating buckling of the ligamentum flavum causing canal narrowing and cord compression in cadavers. Because central hematomyelia of the spinal cord was a consistent finding in postmortem examinations, Schneider concluded that compressive forces were maximal in the central region of the spinal cord resulting in disruption first of gray matter then, with increasing force, involving surrounding white matter; hence his label CCS. Accordingly, medial fibers of the lateral corticospinal tracts adjacent to the gray matter were proposed to be more highly susceptible to injury compared with their lateral counterparts (**Fig. 2**). Schneider hypothesized that lamination of the

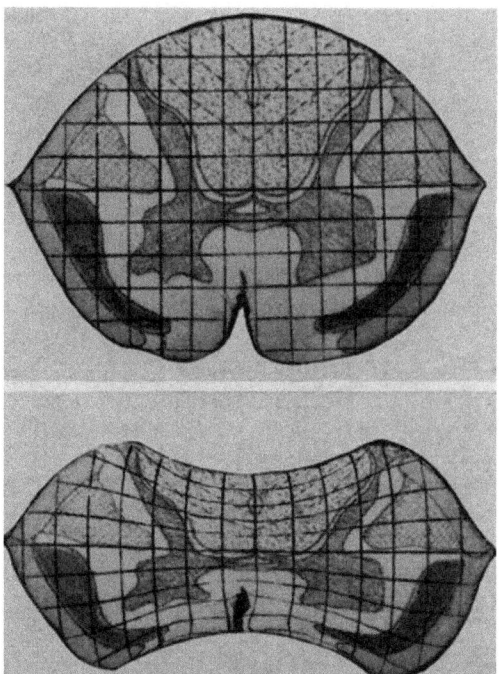

Fig. 2. Schneider's sketches made from a foam model of the cervical spinal cord in cross-section, including major ascending and descending pathways and x- and y-axis grids. (*Top*) Native state with normal anatomy. (*Bottom*) Compressed state from midline anterior osteophytes and posterior ligamentum flavum demonstrating preferential distortion of the central spinal cord with relative sparing of the lateral funiculi. The most medial portion of the corticospinal tract (thought to represent hand function) was proposed to be more selectively compromised than the laterally located leg fibers. (*From* Schneider RC, Cherry G, Pantek H. The syndrome of acute central cervical spinal cord injury; with special reference to the mechanisms involved in hyperextension injuries of cervical spine. *J Neurosurg*. 1954;11(6):546-577. https://doi.org/10.3171/jns.1954.11.6.0546.)

lateral corticospinal tract with hands and arms represented medially was responsible for the clinical findings of the syndrome.[5]

Despite the compelling logic behind Schneider's mechanism, sophisticated axonal labeling experiments and primate spinal cord lesion studies have failed to demonstrate somatotopic organization of the lateral corticospinal tract in the cervical spinal cord.[18,20,21] Indeed based on spinal cord transection studies in primates, the function of the lateral corticospinal tract is to carry motor efferents subserving grasp and hand dexterity rather than global upper and lower limb control.[20,22] Hence in the thoracic spine the corticospinal tract becomes a fraction of the size of its cervical counterpart because it provides more limited input to the legs and digits of the feet.

Further work supports the argument against corticospinal tract lamination. Zheng and colleagues[23] have recently demonstrated significant changes to motor unit activity of lower rather than upper extremity muscles after decompression surgery for CCS. Using histologic techniques in postmortem specimens Bunge and Levi have confirmed the entirety of the lateral corticospinal tracts to be severely affected following central cord injury, not just its medial fibers.[21,22] Meanwhile the ventral corticospinal tract is largely spared, indicating the central and lateral propensity of this injury to involve primarily gray matter and adjacent lateral white matter.

Integrating the previously mentioned evidence, it is likely that preferential sensory and motor hand involvement in CCS arises from a combination of nonspecific damage to: ascending second-order spinothalamic axons decussating through the central gray matter; and descending lateral corticospinal tracts in the immediately adjacent white matter, all primarily involved with hand function. A low-velocity/low-impact hyperextension mechanism not forceful enough to cause fracture/dislocation results in buckling of the ligamentum flavum through the area of maximal cervical lordosis: C4, C5, and C6. The spinal cord is compressed between the ligamentum flavum and anterior disk/osteophytes, narrowing the central canal more than the lateral recess. Maximal compressive force is therefore generated in the midline falling off laterally because of the location of these midline stenotic structures. Hence under low velocity and low impact the contents of the spinal cord are displaced into the less compromised lateral recesses. Less severe injuries affect the central gray matter first resulting in hand numbness. More severe hyperextension results in more severe parenchymal displacement and destruction spreading out radially from the center of the spinal cord and into the adjacent lateral corticospinal tracts causing hand and more proximal upper extremity weakness.

In their original descriptions Thorburn[4] and Schneider and coworkers[5] believed the degree of hematomyelia associated with CCS in postmortem specimens worthy of comment. Although they could not know it at the time, it remains likely that intramedullary hemorrhage plays a significant role in the pathophysiology of CCS. In 1986 Wallace and coworkers[24] elegantly demonstrated the intricate reticular network of arterioles supplying the gray matter of the mammalian cervical spinal cord using colloidal carbon angiography (**Fig. 3**). Using an aneurysm clip method of incomplete SCI (hauntingly reminiscent of the mechanism behind CCS described previously) the disruption

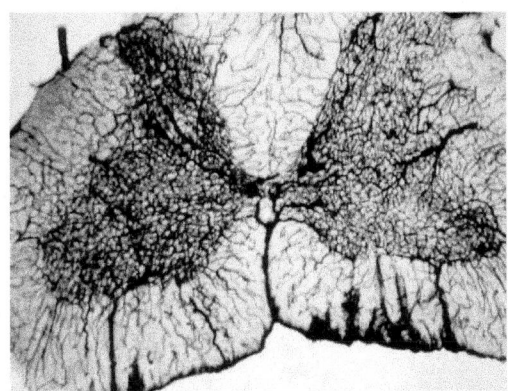

Fig. 3. Colloidal carbon angiogram of a rodent spinal cord taken from the cervical region. Note the fine reticular pattern of the arterioles especially prominent in the gray matter. In contrast to the vertically oriented white matter ascending and descending axons, it is likely that these fragile blood vessels are highly sensitive to stretch and shear with lateral displacement as seen in Figs. 2B, 5, and 6. (*Courtesy of* Dr. Charles H. Tator.)

of the gray matter from intramedullary hemorrhage was striking (**Fig. 4**). In the setting of preexisting spinal stenosis it is easy to imagine shear forces created across these arterioles as they are displaced laterally under midline compression, resulting in disruption and arterial hemorrhage into the gel-like gray matter, expanding laterally into the less stenotic regions of the lateral funiculi (**Fig. 5**).

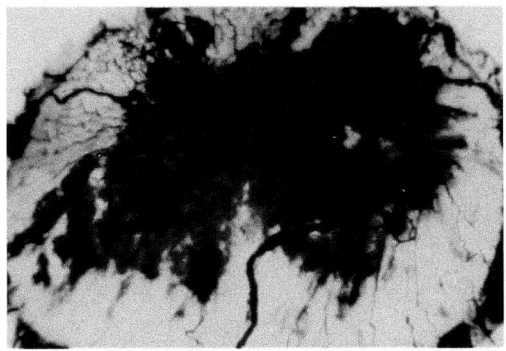

Fig. 4. Colloidal carbon angiogram of a rodent spinal cord subjected to an acute compressive injury using the calibrated aneurysm clip model. Compressive forces are delivered to the anterior and posterior surfaces of the cord when the clip is applied, displacing spinal cord tissue laterally. The strength of this clip was set for an incomplete injury. Note the preference for hemorrhagic transformation in the gray matter with relative preservation of the more peripherally located white matter tracts. (*Courtesy of* Dr. Charles H. Tator.)

In summary the pathophysiology of CCS typically occurs in the setting of preexisting stenosis and involves a low-impact/low-velocity hyperextension injury to the neck. This causes buckling of the ligamentum flavum at the lordotic apex of the cervical spine (C4-C6) resulting in spinal cord compression against osteophytes and disks protruding into the anterior canal, displacing the spinal cord parenchyma into the less stenotic lateral recesses. The epicenter of compression is in the sagittal midline but spreads laterally proportional to the force involved and degree of preexisting stenosis. Spinal cord gray matter is affected first because of stretch and shear to the transversely oriented sensory afferents crossing the midline and the arteriole blood supply; their side-to-side horizontal trajectory makes them more susceptible to damage from lateral displacement than the longitudinally oriented white matter tracts (**Fig. 6**). Gray matter injury results in sensory disturbance to the hands. With higher injury forces shear and contusion extend laterally to involve white matter tracts in a medial-to-lateral preference. Motor weakness of the hands is precipitated from indiscriminate lateral corticospinal pathway involvement. With greater injury force there is additional lateral, anterior, and posterior white matter involvement affecting arm, leg, bowel, and bladder function.

CCS therefore represents a spectrum of sensory and motor deficits affecting the upper extremities first and the lower extremities later depending on the degree of trauma and stenosis. Implicit in this mechanism is the potential to produce a motor and sensory complete SCI without fracture/dislocation, or an American Spinal Injury Association (ASIA) grade A CCS.

MANAGEMENT

Of all the controversies surrounding CCS, the management of incomplete SCI in this setting is one of the most widely debated. In his original narrative, Schneider and coworkers[5] described the surgical management of CCS to be "... contraindicated because spontaneous improvement or complete recovery may occur. Furthermore, operation has actually been known to harm these patients rather than improve them." In the 65 years ensuing since this warning, the philosophy of a more conservative approach toward surgical intervention for CCS continues to be championed and despaired.

Conservative Treatment

As recently as 2019 Divi and colleagues[25] concluded nonoperative conservative care to be the treatment of choice for CCS echoing the

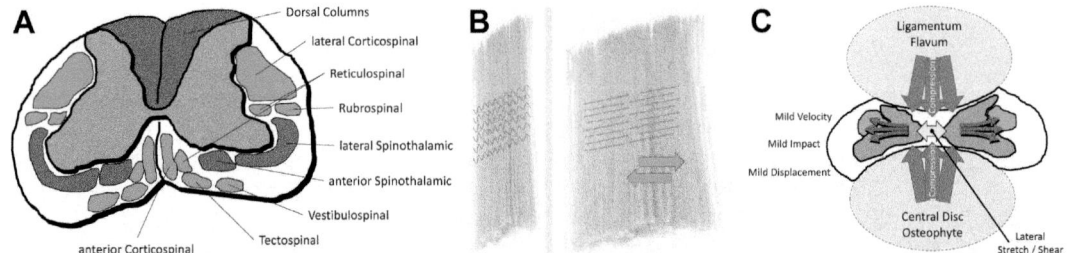

Fig. 5. (*A*) Schematic representation of the major ascending and descending pathways in the human spinal cord and their relationship to the central gray matter. Note the location and size of the lateral corticospinal pathways primarily responsible for hand dexterity, which are much smaller in the thoracic spinal cord. Locomotion has been primarily localized to the more anterior reticulospinal and vestibulospinal pathways. (*B*) Representation (*left*) of ascending and descending white matter axons (spaghetti) in the cervical spinal cord. *Wavy lines* represent horizontally oriented vascular arterioles, interneurons, and segmental somatosensory afferents crossing to ascend in the contralateral spinothalamic tracts. With anterior and posterior compression the vertically oriented axons displace laterally (*right*), with relative immunity while transversely oriented blood vessels and nerves are disproportionately disrupted by stretch and shear. (*C*) Schematic representation of a stenotic spinal canal with overgrown ligamentum flavum and bony osteophyte compressing the spinal cord. Resulting forces displace axons, neurons, glia, and vasculature laterally away from the central compression. This displacement occurs with minor forces compared with traditional fracture dislocation, in many cases sparing peripheral white matter tracts.

original recommendations of Schneider. In 1977 Shrosbree[26] presented a series of 99 patients with cervical spine injuries. In their report 39 patients had hyperextension injuries but the rest were variable with compression fractures and even including two odontoid fractures. Their treatment management consisted of bedrest and immobilization for 12 weeks; facet subluxations were treated with cervical traction in skull tongs.[26] After these conservative measures they found that

from the total of 99 patients, 84% improved to either "Virtually full return; independent (hands slightly involved)" or "Walking with stick; hands more involved."[26] Ishida and Tominaga[27] in 2002 presented a series of 22 patients with CCS in Japan. In their series all patients were treated conservatively with sandbag immobilization for 2 to 3 weeks followed by a cervical collar for 3 to 4 weeks. They found that the most common mechanism of injury was hyperextension. At 2-year

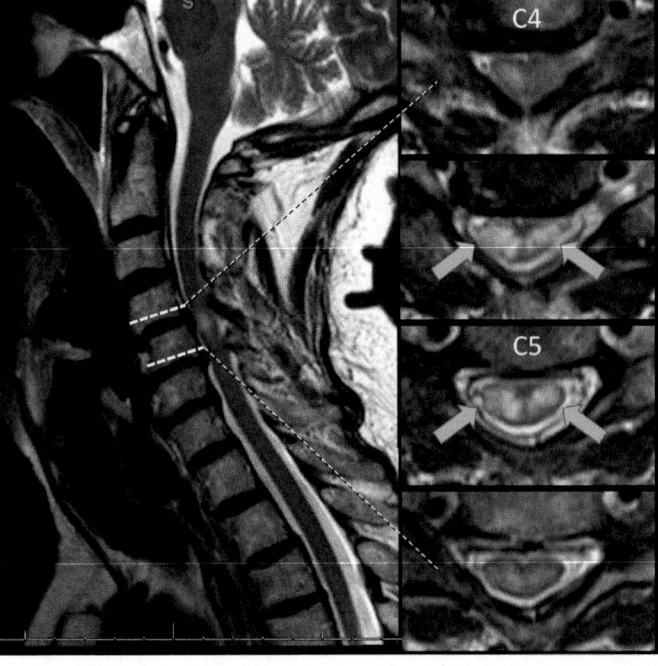

Fig. 6. Sagittal and axial MRI cuts of a patient with post-traumatic CCS in the absence of fracture or dislocation. Pre-existing canal stenosis at the apex of cervical lordosis is apparent. Note abnormal hyperintense signal on the axial images in the gray matter and lateral white matter where the corticospinal tracts are located (*arrows*), sparing anterior and posterior white matter pathways.

follow-up 77% of patients had full motor recovery, and the rest had mild hand dysfunction.[27] Sixty-three percent of patients achieved full recovery in pin prick and light touch at 2 years.[27]

Pollard and Apple[28] in 2003 reviewed more than 20 years of patients with incomplete tetraplegia after cervical SCI at their rehabilitation center. Although their review included 412 patients, they had several missing data points. In particular only 202 patients had complete neurologic examination at the time of injury, which limits some of their findings.[28] Of these patients 97 were diagnosed with CCS, and 57 had SCI in the setting of cervical spine stenosis without fracture or instability. Thirty-eight of these were treated conservatively, whereas 19 underwent surgical decompression. The authors found that there was no difference in neurologic examination 9 days after surgery between the groups. From their large cohort of patients with SCI (412 patients), patients with CCS had an overall improvement of 30 points in the SCI injury scale from initial injury to last follow-up; this represented substantially more improvement compared with the other types of SCI in their case series.[28]

Surgical Treatment

Schneider and coworkers[5,29] reported several of his original patients undergoing extensive laminectomies and dural opening to section the dentate ligament, and noted a high incidence of neurologic deterioration. Despite his initial misgivings, however, national registry data demonstrate a 40% increase in surgical procedures performed for CCS in the last decade, perhaps fueled by improved perioperative care and surgical techniques compared with the 1950s.[30,31]

More recent studies document neurologic recovery in patients treated surgically for CCS.[32–40] Uribe and colleagues[36] evaluated 29 patients with CCS treated with expansile laminoplasty, and reported most (71%) improved by one ASIA grade at 3 months. In a 21-year retrospective review of 126 CSS patients, Stevens and colleagues[39] reported those who received surgical intervention had a statistically significant improvement compared with those treated with medical management alone, gaining at least one grade in the Frankel scale with a mean follow-up of 32 months. Guest and colleagues[40] reviewed their series of 50 patients with CCS; all patients underwent surgical decompression and all improved at least 30 out of 100 points from baseline over a mean follow-up period of 36 months.

Of 49 patients with CCS decompressed acutely by Chen and colleagues[33] all had an improvement in at least 20 points in their ASIA motor scores, whereas those operated within 4 days of injury realized up to 32 points of improvement. Most recovery was noted within 6 months of surgery; follow-up to a mean of 56 months revealed further improvement on average less than 10 points.[33] Song and colleagues[41] in 2005 reviewed a series of 22 patients with CCS without fractures or dislocations who underwent surgical intervention. In their series all patients improved at least one Frankel grade, whereas four patients (18%) improved two grades. Mean time from injury to surgery in the cohort was 8 days. The timing of surgery was determined based on neurologic severity; patients that had early improvement had later surgery compared with those with more profound deficits.[41] This remains a treatment algorithm commonly practiced today.

Timing of Surgery

Perhaps, perhaps even more widely debated than the need for decompressive surgery in CCS, is the timing of surgery. It is generally accepted that incomplete SCI from fracture dislocation should be treated by early decompression and stabilization. However, timing of surgery for incomplete CCS in the absence of acute fracture or dislocation varies widely from one institution and one surgeon to another.[35] Some surgeons prefer to manage their patients weeks or months beyond the acute injury phase after they achieve a neurologic plateau.[42] Evidence is limited and controversy common.

In their series of 126 patients with CCS, Stevens and colleagues[39] found early decompression (<24 hours) and delayed decompression (>24 hours) resulted in motor improvement for the entire cohort; there were no detectable differences in neurologic outcome between the two groups.[39] Chen and colleagues[32] operated on patients with CCS after a mean of 9 days after injury. Their main criteria for surgical treatment was lack of improvement or worsening of neurologic function. They compared their results with patients that were treated nonoperatively and found delayed surgery provided more rapid improvement in motor function; 81% of patients improved immediately after surgery allowing early mobilization, earlier discharge, and shorted periods of rehabilitation.[32] However, this benefit was transient: there was no difference in neurologic outcome between the operative and nonoperative groups at 6 months follow-up.[32]

Guest and colleagues[40] analyzed patients treated less than 24 hours after injury and those greater than 24 hours after injury. They found that patients with fracture dislocation benefitted the most from early surgery, with an average intensive care unit stay 6 days shorter compared with those operated greater than 24 hours. Aarabi and colleagues[43] in 2011 reviewed a case series of 42 patients with CCS without fracture or dislocation, comparing neurologic outcomes between those patients undergoing surgery less than 24 hours from admission, 24 to 48 hours, and greater than 48 hours. Nine patients underwent surgery less than 24 hours, 10 patients within 24 to 48 hours, 17 patients between 3 and 7 days, and 3 patients within 6 weeks. Although all patients improved neurologically at 12 months their results did not show any difference in motor scores between the different timing of surgery.[43]

In summary, although early surgery may benefit patients with severe SCI in the short term by reducing intensive care unit stay, allowing early mobilization, and shortening total hospital stay, the long-term neurologic outcomes of early versus delayed surgery in CCS so far seem to be similar particularly when long-term follow-up is available.[25,32,39] Conversely, surgical decompression of the cervical spinal cord in the acute setting may not be without risk. Reperfusion injuries (white cord syndrome) have been reported after surgical decompression of a stenotic canal resulting in cord re-expansion, increased MRI signal change (hemorrhage), and neurologic deterioration to the point of quadriplegia.[44,45]

Spine society guidelines
Based on much the same evidence as presented above, the American Association of Neurologic Surgeons/Congress of Neurologic Surgeons Joint Guidelines Committee recommends that patients with CCS should have "surgical decompression of the compressed spinal cord, particularly if the compression is focal and anterior."[18] Medical management in the intensive care unit is recommended to monitor hemodynamic parameters and augment the blood pressure for a mean arterial pressure between 85 and 90 mm Hg for up to the first week after injury.[18] They did not find enough evidence to make recommendations on the timing of surgery.

The AO spine guidelines committee proposes that: "early surgery (<24 hours after injury) be considered as a treatment option in adult patients with traumatic central cord syndrome" without evidence of mechanical instability, acknowledging that the quality of the evidence is low, and the strength of the recommendation is weak.[46]

The International Spinal Cord Society recommends that "patients with CCS secondary to an extension injury in a stenotic canal without

fracture/dislocation/instability/disc herniation can be given the options to undergo either surgical management {especially in selected cases with substantial neurologic deficit (AIS C) in the presence of ongoing cord compression} or an initial conservative management followed by surgery at a later date, if there is neurologic deterioration or plateau of neurologic recovery."[47]

In summary, the literature providing evidence for decompression and timing of surgery in patients with CCS is disparate. Current guidelines allow for common sense and surgeon/patient preference. Establishing simple and unequivocal criteria to provide a reliable diagnosis for CCS will enable more robust data on which to base these decisions.

CENTRAL CORD SYNDROME REDEFINED

In almost 70 years since Schneider labeled it CCS, it has been learned that the primary demographic of this injury involves an older population with preexisting cervical stenosis suffering low-velocity/low-impact hyperextension neck trauma without fracture or dislocation. The predisposition of CCS to involve hand sensory and motor function before arm and leg function further argues for unique pathophysiology compared with traditional incomplete SCI. However, the ability to understand and treat this important condition has been hampered by the inability to diagnose it in a reliable and timely manner.

We propose a simplified definition for CCS to include any type of acute sensory or motor deficit localized to the cervical spinal cord from a traumatic event in the absence of fracture or dislocation. Symptoms, such as numbness and tingling in the hands or fingers, returning to normal within 24 hours should still be classified as a spinal cord concussion. However, hand and finger sensory symptoms without motor deficit persisting longer than 24 hours should be considered the mildest form of CCS, triggering referral for neurosurgical or spine surgery evaluation. In its most severe form CCS may present as a complete ASIA grade A SCI localized to the cervical spine without fracture or dislocation.

Ruling out fracture or dislocation should be performed by routine radiograph or preferably spiral computed tomography scan. Nonspecific ligamentous signal change on MR imaging with normal bony alignment should not be accepted as de facto evidence of dislocation. However, a hyperextension injury with anterior longitudinal ligament disruption and disk space widening (± epidural hematoma) would not fit this definition of CCS because of the possibility of temporary dislocation/translation compressing the spinal cord at the time of trauma. In contrast to CCS, SCI without radiographic abnormality (SCIWORA) must be considered in an adolescent or young adult in the setting of high-velocity/high-impact trauma and evidence of ligamentous injury on MRI sequences. CCS might be considered a subset of SCI without evidence of trauma (SCIWORET).[48] However, the definition of SCIWORET embraces a broader more non-specific spectrum of SCI in deference to the pathophysiological considerations described above.

Simplifying the definition of CCS not only helps purify the diagnosis based on pathophysiology but generates more meaningful comparisons between institutional populations locally, nationally, and worldwide, helping future studies better objectify the natural history and outcome from different types of treatment. In addition, this kind of simplicity facilitates the study of CCS in large populations captured by national datasets.

SUMMARY

CCS is the most common type of incomplete SCI. Current epidemiologic trends predict an increasing proportion of the population to become afflicted with this type of injury. Despite Schneider identifying the syndrome more than 60 years ago, heterogeneity in patient populations and diagnostic criteria continues to muddy the current understanding of this condition. As a result, controversies over management persist ranging the entire spectrum of nonsurgical to surgical care. A new, more concise definition of central cord syndrome will allow us to identify it on a national level through registry data, and help future studies to elucidate characteristics and optimize treatment strategies specific to this important and emerging condition.

CLINICS CARE POINTS

- Central cord syndrome (CCS) can present as numbness and tingling in the hands ranging to complete quadriplegia.
- CCS occurs in the setting of low-impact/low-velocity trauma in adults without fracture/dislocation with preexisting cervical spondylosis.
- Provided the patient is stable or improving neurologically, surgical decompression is recommended but can be performed in an elective or semielective manner.

- Patients demonstrating progressive neurologic deterioration should have emergent decompression.

DISCLOSURE

The authors have nothing to disclose.

REFERENCES

1. Diaz E, Morales H. Spinal cord anatomy and clinical syndromes. Semin Ultrasound CT MRI 2016;37(5):360–71.
2. Tattersall R, Turner B. Brown-Séquard and his syndrome. Lancet 2000;356(9223):61–3.
3. Hashmi SZ, Marra A, Jenis LG, et al. Current concepts: central cord syndrome. Clin Spine Surg 2018;31(10):407–12.
4. Thorburn W. Cases of injury to the cervical region of the spinal cord. Brain 1887;9(4):510–43.
5. Schneider RC, Cherry G, Pantek H. The syndrome of acute central cervical spinal cord injury; with special reference to the mechanisms involved in hyperextension injuries of cervical spine. J Neurosurg 1954;11(6):546–77.
6. Bosch A, Stauffer ES, Nickel VL. Incomplete traumatic quadriplegia. A ten-year review. JAMA 1971;216(3):473–8.
7. McKinley W, Santos K, Meade M, et al. Incidence and outcomes of spinal cord injury clinical syndromes. J Spinal Cord Med 2007;30(3):215–24.
8. Lenehan B, Street J, O'Toole P, et al. Central cord syndrome in Ireland: the effect of age on clinical outcome. Eur Spine J 2009;18(10):1458–63.
9. Penrod LE, Hegde SK, Ditunno JF. Age effect on prognosis for functional recovery in acute, traumatic central cord syndrome. Arch Phys Med Rehabil 1990;71(12):963–8.
10. Stevenson CM, Dargan DP, Warnock J, et al. Traumatic central cord syndrome: neurological and functional outcome at 3 years. Spinal Cord 2016;54(11):1010–5.
11. Hagen EM, Eide GE, Rekand T, et al. A 50-year follow-up of the incidence of traumatic spinal cord injuries in Western Norway. Spinal Cord 2010;48(4):313–8.
12. Ahoniemi E, Alaranta H, Hokkinen E-M, et al. Incidence of traumatic spinal cord injuries in Finland over a 30-year period. Spinal Cord 2008;46(12):781–4.
13. Toda M, Nakatani E, Omae K, et al. Age-specific characterization of spinal cord injuries over a 19-year period at a Japanese rehabilitation center. PLoS One 2018;13(3):e0195120.

14. Devivo MJ. Epidemiology of traumatic spinal cord injury: trends and future implications. Spinal Cord 2012;50(5):365–72.

15. Jain NB, Ayers GD, Peterson EN, et al. Traumatic spinal cord injury in the United States, 1993-2012. JAMA 2015;313(22):2236–43.

16. University of Alabama. National Spinal Cord Injury Statistical Center, facts and figures at a glance 2019. Available at: https://www.nscisc.uab.edu/Public/Facts%20and%20Figures%202019%20-%20Final.pdf.

17. DeVivo MJ, Chen Y. Trends in new injuries, prevalent cases, and aging with spinal cord injury. Arch Phys Med Rehabil 2011;92(3):332–8.

18. Aarabi B, Hadley MN, Dhall SS, et al. Management of acute traumatic central cord syndrome (ATCCS). Neurosurgery 2013;72(suppl_3):195–204.

19. Taylor AR. The mechanism of injury to the spinal cord in the neck without damage to vertebral column. J Bone Joint Surg Br 1951;33-B(4):543–7.

20. Levi AD, Tator CH, Bunge RP. Clinical syndromes associated with disproportionate weakness of the upper versus the lower extremities after cervical spinal cord injury. Neurosurgery 1996;38(1):179–83 [discussion 183-185].

21. Jimenez O, Marcillo A, Levi AD. A histopathological analysis of the human cervical spinal cord in patients with acute traumatic central cord syndrome. Spinal Cord 2000;38(9):532–7.

22. Bunge RP, Puckett WR, Becerra JL, et al. Observations on the pathology of human spinal cord injury. A review and classification of 22 new cases with details from a case of chronic cord compression with extensive focal demyelination. Adv Neurol 1993;59:75–89.

23. Zheng C, Yu Q, Shan X, et al. Early surgical decompression ameliorates dysfunction of spinal motor neuron in patients with acute traumatic central cord syndrome: an ambispective cohort analysis. Spine 2020;45(14):E829–38.

24. Wallace MC, Tator CH, Frazee P. Relationship between posttraumatic ischemia and hemorrhage in the injured rat spinal cord as shown by colloidal carbon angiography. Neurosurgery 1986;18(4):433–9.

25. Divi SN, Schroeder GD, Mangan JJ, et al. Management of acute traumatic central cord syndrome: a narrative review. Glob Spine J 2019;9(1 Suppl):89S–97S.

26. Shrosbree RD. Acute central cervical spinal cord syndrome: aetiology, age incidence and relationship to the orthopaedic injury. Paraplegia 1977;14(4):251–8.

27. Ishida Y, Tominaga T. Predictors of neurologic recovery in acute central cervical cord injury with only upper extremity impairment. Spine (Phila Pa 1976) 2002;27(15):1652–8 [discussion 1658].

28. Pollard ME, Apple DF. Factors associated with improved neurologic outcomes in patients with incomplete tetraplegia. Spine (Phila Pa 1976) 2003;28(1):33–9.

29. Schneider RC. A syndrome in acute cervical spine injuries for which early operation is indicated. J Neurosurg 1951;8(4):360–7.

30. Brodell DW, Jain A, Elfar JC, et al. National trends in the management of central cord syndrome: an analysis of 16,134 patients. Spine J 2015;15(3):435–42.

31. Yoshihara H, Yoneoka D. Trends in the treatment for traumatic central cord syndrome without bone injury in the United States from 2000 to 2009. J Trauma Acute Care Surg 2013;75(3):453–8.

32. Chen TY, Dickman CA, Eleraky M, et al. The role of decompression for acute incomplete cervical spinal cord injury in cervical spondylosis. Spine 1998;23(22):2398–403.

33. Chen L, Yang H, Yang T, et al. Effectiveness of surgical treatment for traumatic central cord syndrome. J Neurosurg Spine 2009;10(1):3–8.

34. Chen TY, Lee ST, Lui TN, et al. Efficacy of surgical treatment in traumatic central cord syndrome. Surg Neurol 1997;48(5):435–40 [discussion 441].

35. Dvorak MF, Fisher CG, Hoekema J, et al. Factors predicting motor recovery and functional outcome after traumatic central cord syndrome: a long-term follow-up. Spine (Phila Pa 1976) 2005;30(20):2303–11.

36. Uribe J, Green BA, Vanni S, et al. Acute traumatic central cord syndrome: experience using surgical decompression with open-door expansile cervical laminoplasty. Surg Neurol 2005;63(6):505–10 [discussion 510].

37. Kepler CK, Kong C, Schroeder GD, et al. Early outcome and predictors of early outcome in patients treated surgically for central cord syndrome. J Neurosurg Spine 2015;23(4):490–4.

38. Koyanagi I, Iwasaki Y, Hida K, et al. Acute cervical cord injury without fracture or dislocation of the spinal column. J Neurosurg 2000;93(1 Suppl):15–20.

39. Stevens EA, Marsh R, Wilson JA, et al. A review of surgical intervention in the setting of traumatic central cord syndrome. Spine J 2010;10(10):874–80.

40. Guest J, Eleraky MA, Apostolides PJ, et al. Traumatic central cord syndrome: results of surgical management. J Neurosurg 2002;97(1 Suppl):25–32.

41. Song J, Mizuno J, Nakagawa H, et al. Surgery for acute subaxial traumatic central cord syndrome without fracture or dislocation. J Clin Neurosci 2005;12(4):438–43.

42. Lenehan B, Fisher CG, Vaccaro A, et al. The urgency of surgical decompression in acute central cord injuries with spondylosis and without instability. Spine (Phila Pa 1976) 2010;35(21 Suppl):S180–6.

43. Aarabi B, Alexander M, Mirvis SE, et al. Predictors of outcome in acute traumatic central cord syndrome due to spinal stenosis. J Neurosurg Spine 2011;14(1):122–30.

44. Mathkour M, Werner C, Riffle J, et al. Reperfusion "white cord" syndrome in cervical spondylotic myelopathy: does mean arterial pressure goal make a difference? Additional case and literature review. World Neurosurg 2020;137:194–9.

45. Seichi A, Takeshita K, Kawaguchi H, et al. Postoperative expansion of intramedullary high-intensity areas on T2-weighted magnetic resonance imaging after cervical laminoplasty. Spine (Phila Pa 1976) 2004;29(13):1478–82 [discussion 1482].

46. Fehlings MG, Tetreault LA, Wilson JR, et al. A clinical practice guideline for the management of patients with acute spinal cord injury and central cord syndrome: recommendations on the timing (≤24 hours versus >24 hours) of decompressive surgery. Glob Spine J 2017;7(3_suppl):195S–202S.

47. Yelamarthy PKK, Chhabra HS, Vaccaro A, et al. Management and prognosis of acute traumatic cervical central cord syndrome: systematic review and Spinal Cord Society-Spine Trauma Study Group position statement. Eur Spine J 2019;28(10):2390–407.

48. Tator CH. Clinical manifestations of acute spinal cord injury. In Benzel EC and Tator CH - Contemporary Management of Spinal Cord Injury, Neurosurgical Topics 1995. pp 15-26.

Section II: Emerging Therapies

Acute, Severe Traumatic Spinal Cord Injury
Monitoring from the Injury Site and Expansion Duraplasty

Samira Saadoun, PhD[a],*, Marios C. Papadopoulos, MD, FRCS(SN)[b]

KEYWORDS

- Blood pressure • Critical care • Decompression • Duraplasty • Intraspinal pressure • Microdialysis
- Spinal cord injury • Spinal cord perfusion pressure

INTRODUCTION

This review focuses on 2 promising management options for acute, severe traumatic spinal cord injury (SCI): monitoring from the injury site and expansion duraplasty. Injury site monitoring for SCI is analogous to injury site monitoring for traumatic brain injury (TBI). We discuss how our understanding of SCI has evolved and introduce novel concepts identified by monitoring from the injured cord. We apply these concepts to answer questions regarding management with emphasis on duraplasty as a novel treatment.

HISTORY

In the Edwin Smith papyrus (ca. 3000 BC), the ancient Egyptians advocated conservative management for patients with SCI who had limb paralysis because their outcome was universally fatal.[1] Hippocrates (ca. 460–370 BC) attempted to reduce the fractured spine using traction devices,[2] whereas Paul of Aegena (ca. 626–690 AD) performed laminectomy using wine to wash the wound and compression dressings to control bleeding.[3] The nineteenth century London surgeon Astley Cooper carried out decompressions for SCI.[4] He often operated with no warning; many of his patients were terrified and refused to consent, but Cooper believed that it was the surgeon's duty to "get the job done." The dismal results of such operations led the nineteenth century Scottish surgeon/neurologist Charles Bell to propose that all of the cord damage happens at the time of injury rendering ongoing cord compression irrelevant; he concluded that surgical decompression was both dangerous and useless.[4] Bell realized that death after SCI was caused by retention of urine resulting in renal damage and sepsis. This was a major milestone in the treatment of SCI, and Bell's views became widely accepted. Donald Munro (1889–1973) in Boston emphasized the importance of not only managing urinary retention, but also preventing pressure ulcers, treating chest infections, and immobilizing patients to limit deformity.[4,5] During his period at Stoke Mandeville Hospital in the United Kingdom, Ludwig Guttman (1899–1980) formulated the following guidelines: patients should be cared for in specialized units, receive immediate attention by appropriate specialists, undergo continuous monitoring of multiple body systems with thorough documentation, be provided with appropriate aftercare including rehabilitation and vocational retraining, all under the jurisdiction of the public health service and with the cooperation of the Ministry of Pensions and employer.[4,5] Guttman emphasized motivating patients and founded the Paralympics. His integrated treatment program became the mainstay of SCI management in the mid to late twentieth

[a] Academic Neurosurgery Unit, St. George's, University of London, Cranmer Terrace, London SW17 0RE, UK;
[b] Department of Neurosurgery, Atkinson Morley Wing, St. George's Hospital NHS Foundation Trust, Blackshaw Road, London SW17 0QT, UK
* Corresponding author.
E-mail address: ssaadoun@sgul.ac.uk

Neurosurg Clin N Am 32 (2021) 365–376
https://doi.org/10.1016/j.nec.2021.03.008

century, refocusing priorities to psychological rehabilitation and prolonged survival while shifting the emphasis away from surgery. However, over the past 40 years, surgery has regained popularity in attempts to mitigate secondary injury by rapid decompression.[6–8] The effect of early decompression on neurologic outcome remains difficult to quantify.

LESSONS FROM TRAUMATIC BRAIN INJURY

Because the brain and spinal cord are composed of the same cell types, SCI must share common pathologic mechanisms with TBI. Techniques for invasive monitoring in the setting of TBI have evolved to allow for quantification of intracranial pressure (ICP), cerebral perfusion pressure (CPP), and autoregulation.[9,10] CPP is the pressure driving blood flow to the brain. Autoregulation provides for constant cerebral blood flow (CBF) regardless of CPP. In the normal state this provides a continuous supply of oxygen and the brain's main energy substrate: glucose.

After TBI, the brain swells against the nonexpansile dura and skull. Initially, compensatory mechanisms (reduction in intracranial venous and cerebrospinal fluid [CSF] volumes) buffer rise in ICP. As the compensatory mechanisms become exhausted, autoregulation fails, ICP rises, and CPP falls (Monro-Kellie doctrine). Thus, CBF decreases, causing drop in brain tissue oxygen (PbtO$_2$) and glucose.

In patients suffering severe TBI, ICP is monitored using an intraparenchymal pressure probe and mean arterial blood pressure (MAP) is obtained by an indwelling arterial catheter. This allows the CPP to be calculated (CPP = MAP – ICP).[11] Tissue metabolites and PbtO$_2$ may be monitored using a microdialysis (MD) catheters[12] and an tissue oxygen electrode, respecitively.[11] It is possible to apply these same concepts and techniques to the injured spinal cord, substituting spinal cord perfusion pressure (SCPP) for CPP, intraspinal pressure (ISP) for ICP, and spinal cord tissue oxygen partial pressure (PsctO$_2$) rather than PbtO$_2$.

MONITORING FROM THE INJURY SITE IN SPINAL CORD INJURY
Intraspinal Pressure

After severe SCI, intraspinal pressure (ISP) may be monitored by surgically implanting an intradural extramedullary pressure transducer at the injury site (Fig. 1).[13–15] The ISP signal has interesting properties:

1. At the injury site, subdural ISP is comparable to intraparenchymal pressure.

2. Normal ISP is comparable to ICP with 3 peaks (P1 percussion, P2 tidal, P3 dicrotic) and comparable Fourier transforms (prominent cardiac/respiratory components).
3. ISP at the injury site is higher than ISP above or below.
4. As ISP rises, ISP pulse amplitude also rises and P2 rises above P1 or P3.

These ISP properties support the notion that at the injury site the cord swells circumferentially, initially displacing CSF and ultimately becoming compressed against dura. Spinal cord swelling against the dura after SCI is also evident on MRI[16] and can be conceptualized as resulting in 4 discrete compartments: (1) CSF above; (2) CSF below; (3) injury site; and (4) extradural compartment (Fig. 2).[17] This explains why ISP cannot be reliably determined by monitoring lumbar CSF pressure and why ISP is not effectively reduced by draining CSF.[18] Within its fluctuations, the ISP signal contains "hidden information" about the injury site that may be revealed by a visibility graph analysis[19] and nonlinear dynamic[20] signal analysis.

Risks of Intraspinal Pressure Monitoring

Based on a series of 42 patients with SCI with American Spinal Injury Association Impairment Scale (AIS) grades A to C (Table 1),[21] the most common complications of ISP monitoring are CSF-related, and either spontaneously resolve or can be managed manage by adding extra sutures to the wound. No adverse neurologic events have been reported.

Spinal Cord Perfusion Pressure

SCPP is a more accurate way to monitor cord perfusion at the injury site rather than making inferences from MAP. This argument is analogous to using CPP rather than MAP in TBI. The widespread use of MAP to manage patients with SCI arises because of the invasive nature of measuring ISP requiring surgical access including durotomy for implantation. There have been attempts to monitor ISP via a lumbar CSF catheter.[22,23] Although inserting a lumbar catheter is technically simpler than placing probes at the injury site, in SCI lumbar CSF pressure differs from ISP as the injured cord is compressed against dura.[18] Ideally, the current guidelines of maintaining MAP at 85 to 90 mm Hg for 7 days after SCI[24] should be replaced by SCPP guidelines, which would better reflect degree of spinal cord swelling and local (rather than systemic) perfusion. As can be surmised from the formula SCPP = MAP – ISP, SCPP may be increased by adjusting inotrope dose to increase the MAP.[13]

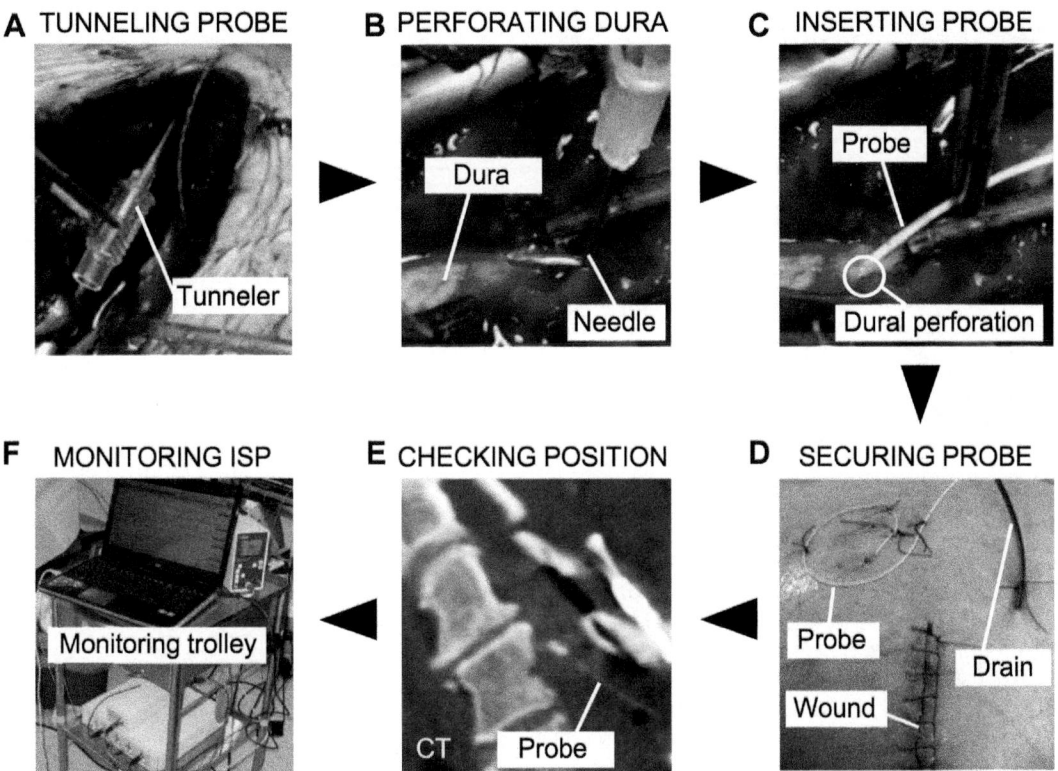

Fig. 1. Monitoring setup. (*A*) A tunneler pulls the pressure probe through the skin into the wound. (*B*) The dura is perforated with a 90° bent needle one level below the injury. (*C*) The pressure probe is inserted through the dural perforation. (*D*) The incision is closed and the probe is secured to skin. (*E*) Computed tomography checks probe position. (*F*) Monitoring trolley kept behind patient bed in ICU. Trolley carries laptop, ICP box, and monitoring system. (*From* Werndle MC, Saadoun S, Phang I et al. Monitoring of spinal cord perfusion pressure in acute spinal cord injury: initial findings of the injured spinal cord pressure evaluation study. Crit Care Med 2014;42(3):646-55; with permission.)

Implications for Wound Care

Laminectomies in patients with SCI with a swollen spinal cord compressed against dura allow easy transmission of external forces to the spinal cord. External compression of the wound leads to increased pressure within the spinal cord, causing potentially catastrophic rise in ISP and fall in SCPP (**Fig. 3**).[13,21] Placing gauze pads on either side of the wound or including cross-links in the rod–pedicle screw construct may prevent external forces from compressing the injured cord.

FOUR COMPARTMENTS

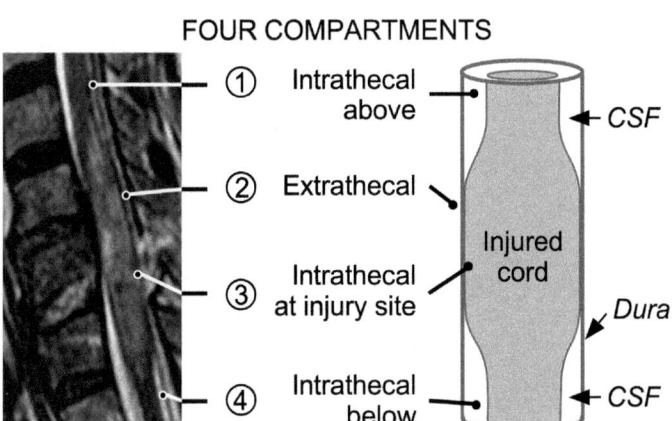

① Intrathecal above

② Extrathecal

③ Intrathecal at injury site

④ Intrathecal below

CSF

Injured cord

Dura

CSF

Fig. 2. Compartmentalization after SCI. MRI (*left*) and schematic (*right*) of the 4 compartments that form after SCI. 1. Intrathecal above injury, 2. Extrathecal, 3. Intrathecal at injury site (cord compressed against dura), 4. Intrathecal below injury. (*Adapted from* Papadopoulos MC. Intrathecal Pressure After Spinal Cord Injury. Neurosurgery 2015;77(3):E500; with permission.)

Table 1
Risks of intraspinal pressure monitoring from the injury site

Complication	Patients		Comments
	No.	%	
Cerebrospinal fluid leak	3/42	7	Resolved by wound resuturing
Wound infection or breakdown	0/42	0	
Meningitis (septic)	0/42	0	
Pseudomeningocele	8/42	19	All resolved at 6-month MRI
Probe displacement	1/42	2	
Neurologic deterioration	0/42	0	
Hematoma	0/42	0	

For further discussion of complications see Ref.[21]

OPTIMIZING CORD PERFUSION

A consequence of spinal cord swelling against the nonelastic dura is that spinal cord tissue must obey the Monro-Kellie doctrine with a pressure-volume relation analogous to that of brain,[15] that is, exhaustion of compensatory reserve and loss of autoregulation as the tissue swells. The more impaired the spinal cord, the more deranged its autoregulation. In TBI, autoregulation may be quantified using the pressure reactivity index PRx (running correlation coefficient between ISP and MAP); we term the corresponding SCI parameter spinal PRx (sPRx). sPRx ≤ 0 indicates intact autoregulation and sPRx greater than 0 deranged autoregulation.[13,25] sPRx rises as ISP increases; that is, as the cord swells, autoregulation is lost.[13] The sPRx versus SCPP relationship is U-shaped (**Fig. 4**A); the ideal goal is for an SCPP that optimizes autoregulation, termed $SCPP_{opt}$. Thus, monitoring and analysis of the sPRx versus

SCPP curve allows determination of $SCPP_{opt}$ and suggests it generally to be 80 - 90 mm Hg.

Cord Hyperperfusion May Be Detrimental

As SCPP decreases below $SCPP_{opt}$, autoregulation is deranged due to cord ischemia. Interestingly, as SCPP increases above $SCPP_{opt}$, autoregulation is also impaired, which suggests that cord hyperperfusion is also detrimental.[13] The mechanism by which hyperperfusion impairs cord function is unknown but possibilities include the following:

1. *Steal phenomenon.* Hyperperfusion increases overall spinal cord blood flow (SCBF), but heterogeneously: well-perfused regions become more perfused whereas underperfused regions become less perfused.[26]
2. *Cord edema.* Hyperperfusion may exacerbate cord edema at the injury site.

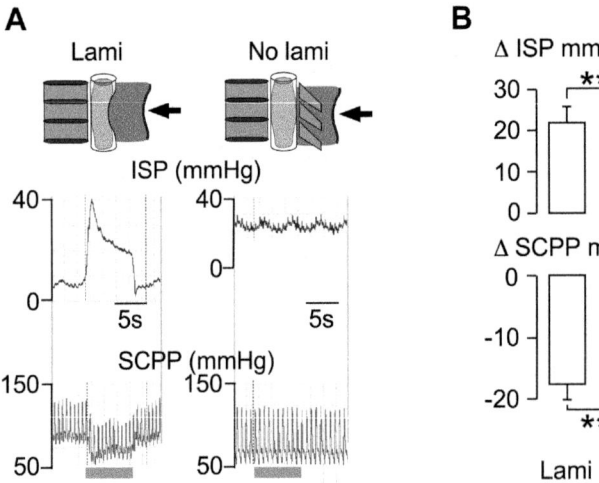

Fig. 3. Effect of wound compression on ISP and SCPP. (*A*) Compressing skin incision in (*left*) laminectomized (Lami) and (*right*) non-laminectomized (No lami) patients with corresponding ISP and SCPP traces. (*B*) ΔISP and ΔSCPP from wound compression (Lami n = 10, No lami n = 7). Mean ± standard error, ***P<0.001. (*Adapted from* Werndle MC, Saadoun S, Phang I et al. Monitoring of spinal cord perfusion pressure in acute spinal cord injury: initial findings of the injured spinal cord pressure evaluation study*. Crit Care Med 2014;42(3):646-55; with permission.)

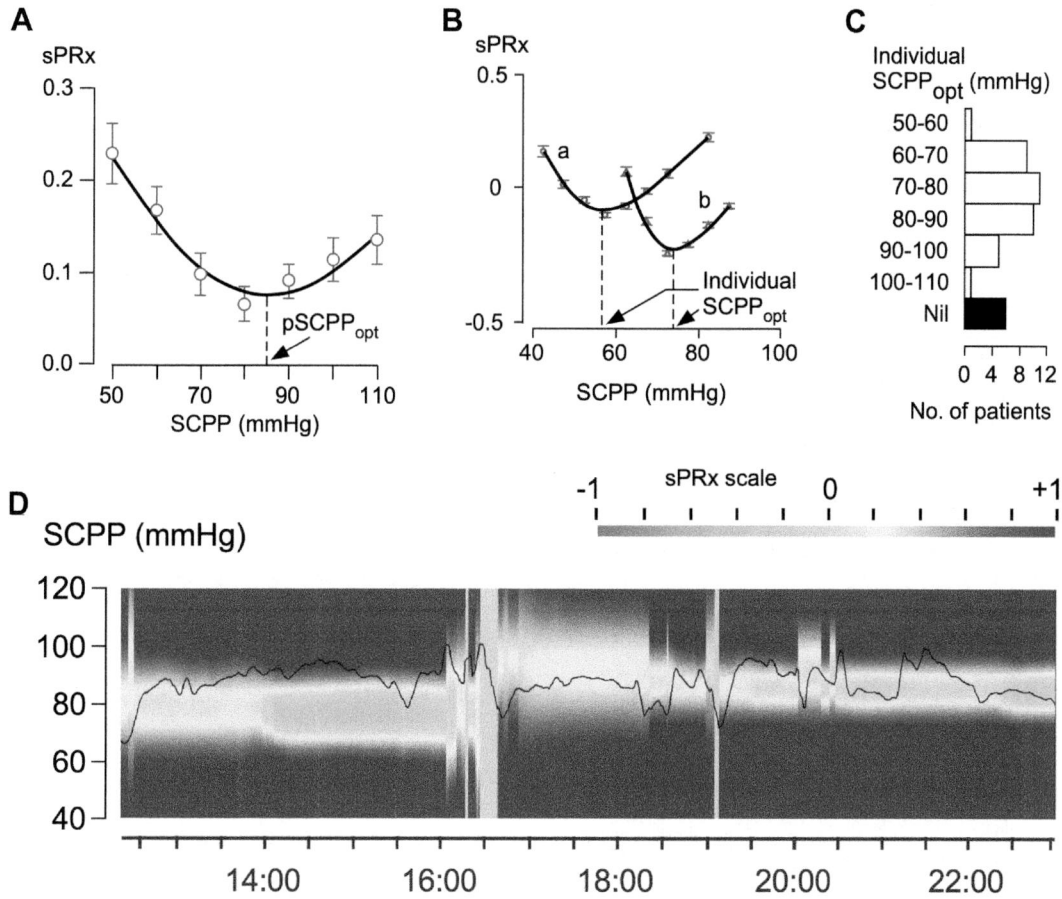

Fig. 4. $SCPP_{opt}$ concept. (*A*) sPRx versus SCPP using pooled data from 45 patients. Dotted line shows pooled $SCPP_{opt}$. (*B*) sPRx versus SCPP for 2 patients (a, b). Dotted line shows each patient's $SCPP_{opt}$ computed from the entire monitoring period. (*C*) Individual $SCPP_{opt}$ values for 45 patients. Nil: $SCPP_{opt}$ not computable. Mean ± standard error. (*D*) Continuous SCPP versus time. sPRx zones: Red (loss of autoregulation), Green (preserved autoregulation), and Yellow (transition from preserved to impaired autoregulation). Line is actual SCPP. (*Adapted from* Chen S, Smielewski P, Czosnyka M et al. Continuous Monitoring and Visualization of Optimum Spinal Cord Perfusion Pressure in Patients with Acute Cord Injury. J Neurotrauma 2017;34(21):2941-9; with permission.)

3. *Cord hemorrhage.* Hyperperfusion may cause hemorrhages in the injured cord.

Individualized Management

Fig. 4B shows sPRx versus SCPP plots for 2 patients (rather than the pooled patient data in **Fig. 4**A). Interestingly, $SCPP_{opt}$ varies widely between patients(**Fig. 4**C),[27] which leads to the concept of individualized management based on $SCPP_{opt}$. $SCPP_{opt}$ is likely influenced by several factors that vary between patients, including the extent of damage to spinal cord and blood vessels, preexisting conditions (hypertension, smoking, diabetes) and the level of injury (because some sites require lower SCBF than others). The concept of individualized $SCPP_{opt}$ may be refined

further.[27] First, it is likely there is a range of physiologic SCPPs with intact autoregulation, that is, $SCPP_{opt}$ is a range not a single value. Second, $SCPP_{opt}$ may vary with time in each patient. The latter argues for continuous $SCPP_{opt}$ monitoring, computed and updated every minute (**Fig. 4**D).

MICRODIALYSIS MONITORING

In addition to invasive ISP monitoring, additional probes may be positioned inside the dura to monitor the partial pressure of oxygen in spinal cord tissue ($PsctO_2$) and to sample interstitial fluid by microdialysis (MD)[28] (**Fig. 5**). MD catheters placed on the surface of an organ provide similar readings as intraparenchymal catheters for pig heart,[29] liver,[30] esophagus,[31] and small bowel.[32]

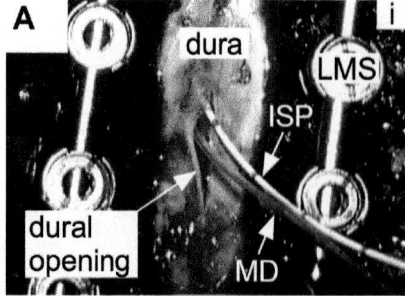

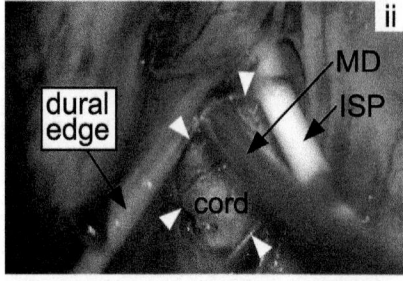

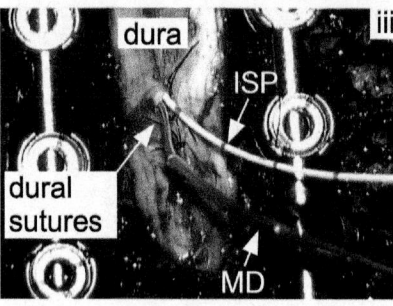

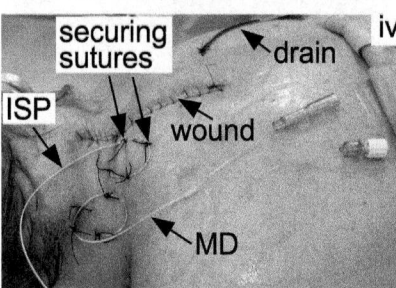

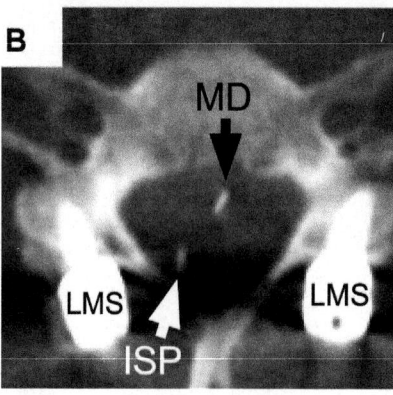

Fig. 5. MD monitoring at injury site. (*A*) i. Insertion of ISP probe and MD catheter under dura and arachnoid.

We thus elected to place the MD catheter on the surface of the injured cord, under the dura and the arachnoid membranes.[28]

The metabolic changes detected by a MD catheter at the injury site correlates with injury severity, SCPP, and injury site metabolism.[28,33] Inserting 2 MD catheters, one at the injury site and another below, provides markedly different metabolic profiles; the distal catheter of course demonstrating more normal metabolism than the injury site catheter.[17,28,33] These studies indicate that MD monitoring from the injury site is feasible and may provide important information about injury metabolism amenable to intervention.

Information from Microdialysis Monitoring

Below, we illustrate how MD may be useful:

1. *Fever.* Most patients with SCI develop fever early after injury.[17] Data obtained from 759 hours of MD monitoring in 44 patients with SCI revealed that fever is associated with metabolic stress at the injury site.[17] The fever burden in the first 2 weeks after SCI predicts AIS grade improvement, independent of other prognosticators, validated in 2 SCI patient cohorts from different centers. Thus, the hypothesis that eliminating fever improves neurologic outcome merits further investigation.

2. *Hypothermia.* We used MD monitoring to determine the impact on the injured cord of local hypothermia in 5 patients with acute, severe thoracic SCI.[34] Cooling altered injury site metabolism (increased tissue glucose, lactate, Lactate/Pyruvate Ratio (LPR), glutamate; decreased glycerol) and reduced cord inflammation (reduced tissue interleukin [IL]-1β, IL-8, monocyte chemoattractant protein [MCP], macrophage inflammatory protein [MIP]1α, MIP1β). Compared with the precooling baseline, rewarming significantly worsened cord physiology (increased ISP, decreased SCPP), metabolism (increased lactate, LPR; decreased glucose, glycerol) and inflammation (increased IL-1β, IL-8, IL-4, IL-10, MCP, MIP1α). We concluded that, after SCI, hypothermia was potentially beneficial by reducing cord

---

ii. Magnified view of dural entry site. Arrowheads show arachnoid. iii. Sutured dural entry site. iv. Prone patient with cervical SCI at end of surgery. LMS, lateral mass screw. (*B*) Postoperative computed tomography scan of cervical spine. (*Adapted from* Phang I, Zoumprouli A, Papadopoulos MC et al. Microdialysis to Optimize Cord Perfusion and Drug Delivery in Spinal Cord Injury. Ann Neurol 2016;80(4):522-31; with permission.)

inflammation, but rewarming was detrimental because of increased cord swelling, ischemia, and inflammation.

3. *Pharmacotherapy.* We administered a bolus of dexamethasone intravenously to 3 patients with SCI and monitored its concentration in the serum and injury site microdialysate. Increasing SCPP by approximately 10 mm Hg increased the entry of dexamethasone into the injury cord approximately threefold, suggesting roles for both MD and SCPP in optimizing drug delivery to the injury site.[28]

4. *Clinical trials.* The preceding findings suggest that ISP and MD monitoring from the injury site may aid randomized controlled trials (RCTs) examining hypothermia/rewarming[34] and neuroprotective drugs.[28] One needs to first determine conditions that maximize benefits and minimize adverse effects of hypothermia/rewarming on cord metabolism and inflammation, for example, by slowing the rewarm speed, and to optimize drug penetration at the injury site. Such monitoring was not part of NABIS II,[35] Cool Kids,[36] or EuroTherm[37] that evaluated hypothermia/rewarming in TBI, or of the National Acute Spinal Cord Injury Study,[38] that evaluated methylprednisolone in SCI.

INJURY SITE MONITORING AND OUTCOME

Although definitive proof to establish that injury site monitoring improves outcome may depend on RCTs, mounting evidence suggests that ISP and SCPP directed management may be beneficial:

1. *Correlations.* In 45 patients with SCI with AIS grade A to C, there was strong correlation between mean ISP and mean SCPP on admission with long-term neurologic improvement.[39] Patients with AIS C SCI exhibited strong correlations between fluctuations in ISP and SCPP, and variations in limb motor scores in the first week after injury.[13,39]

2. *Intervention to increase SCPP.* Increasing SCPP in some patients improves the amplitude of motor evoked responses at or below the injury site,[13] limb motor score,[13] sensory level,[40] and urinary function (manuscript in preparation).

3. *Causality analysis.* Establishing causation in medicine is based on the totality of evidence that includes strong association, biological mechanism, consistency of findings, temporal sequence, and dose-response.[41] Clive Granger developed a mathematical definition of causality based on the notion that causes precede and help predict effect.[42] To test the hypothesis that increasing SCPP improves limb motor score, we considered the time series SCPP versus time and limb motor score versus time. We first used earlier limb motor scores to predict future limb motor scores. Then, we used earlier limb motor scores plus earlier SCPP values to predict future limb motor scores. If the inclusion of earlier SCPP values improves the prediction of future limb motor scores, compared with using earlier limb motor scores alone, then SCPP Granger causes limb motor score. Granger analysis applied to 19 patients with AIS grade C SCI, revealed causal relations among ICP, SCPP, LPR, and limb motor score, summarized in **Fig. 6**.[43]

EXPANSION DURAPLASTY
Reducing Intraspinal Pressure May Be Beneficial

An alternative to increasing SCPP after SCI (by augmenting MAP using inotropes) is to reduce ISP, which may be equally or perhaps even more beneficial:

1. *Increased SCPP.* Because SCPP = MAP – ISP, reducing ISP increases SCPP.

2. *Reduced inotrope requirements.* Reducing ISP means lower MAP achieves the same SCPP, thus reducing inotrope requirements. Inotropes cause cardiogenic complications in SCI, especially in patients older than 60 years.[44,45]

3. *Shorter stay in intensive care unit (ICU).* In an MRI study of 65 patients with SCI, dural cord

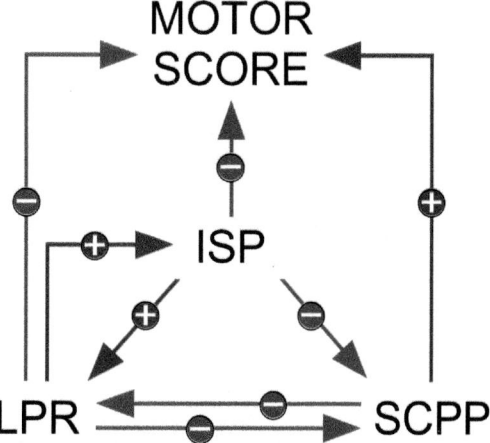

Fig. 6. Granger causality relations in SCI. Each arrow indicates the direction of information flow, that is, causal influence. "+" or "−" indicate the correlation between the variables. For further details of about causality analysis see Ref.[43]

compression resolved slowly ($t_{1/2}$ ~9 days),[16] that is, without ISP reduction, patients with SCI require prolonged ICU stay to optimize SCPP. Reducing ISP may thus reduce ICU stay.

4. *High ISP may be detrimental.* The higher the ISP, the more impaired spinal cord autoregulation becomes,[13,15] and at least theoretically, the higher the risk of blood vessel rupture and intraparenchymal hemorrhage.

Reducing partial pressure of arterial CO_2 or administering intravenous mannitol, reduces ICP in TBI but has no impact on ISP in SCI[13]; only expansion duraplasty is known to reduce ISP.[46]

Expansion Duraplasty

Duraplasty involves opening the dorsal dura longitudinally and suturing an elliptical patch of artificial dura to the dural edge (**Fig. 7**), aiming to increase the space around the injured cord to reduce ISP and enhance cord perfusion. Several lines of evidence suggest that expansion duraplasty may be beneficial after SCI:

1. *Exploratory studies:* We assessed the effect of duraplasty on ISP and SCPP after SCI.[46] Compared with bony decompression in 11 patients, bony plus dural decompression in 10 patients reduced ISP by ~10 mm Hg and increased SCPP by ~15 mm Hg. The injured cord expanded into the additional intradural space that had been created by the duraplasty. Beneficial effects of duraplasty after SCI have also been reported in another study.[47] This may be considered analogous to fasciotomies for compartment syndrome in traumatized limbs.

2. *ISP monitoring.* A key finding in our injury site monitoring studies, is that ISP remains high with low SCPP even after antero-posterior bony decompression,[13,48] thus suggesting the dura as a source of ongoing cord compression.

3. *MRI scans.* In 65 patients with SCI without bony compression, dural restriction was evident on

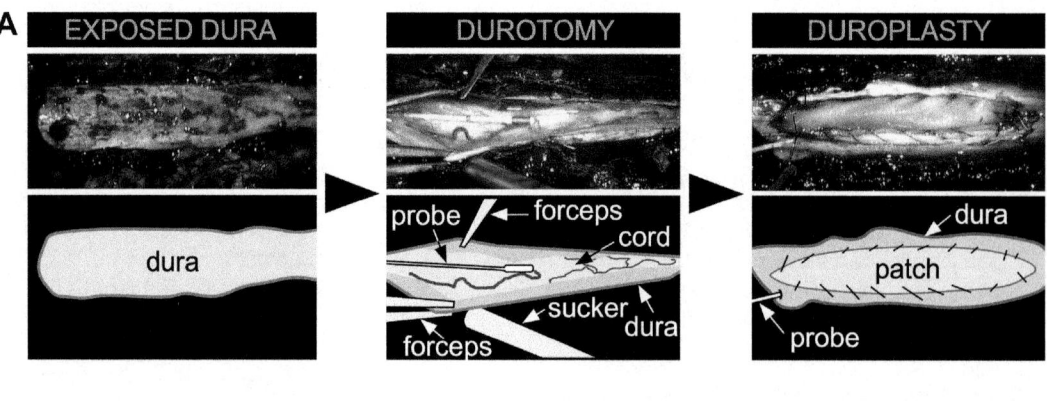

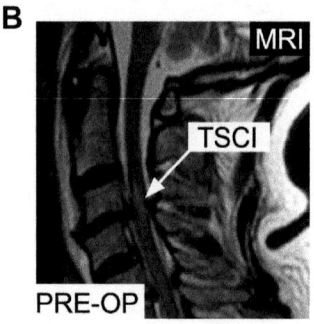
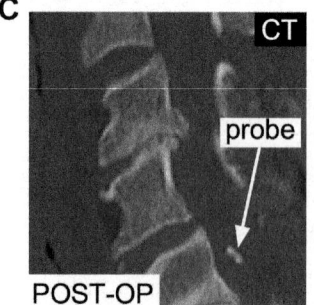
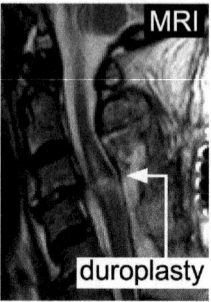

Fig. 7. Expansion duraplasty for SCI. (*A*) (*Left*) Exposed dura after laminectomy. (*Middle*) Durotomy held open with forceps showing injured spinal cord and ISP probe. (*Right*) Sutured dural patch. (*B*) Preoperative T2 MRI showing high signal at site of SCI. (*C*) Postoperative (*left*) Computed tomography showing ISP probe and (*right*) T2 MRI showing duraplasty. (*Adapted from* Phang I, Werndle MC, Saadoun S et al. Expansion duraplasty improves intraspinal pressure, spinal cord perfusion pressure, and vascular pressure reactivity index in patients with traumatic spinal cord injury: injured spinal cord pressure evaluation study. J Neurotrauma 2015;32(12):865-74; with permission.)

Table 2
Complications of expansion duraplasty for spinal cord injury

Complication	No.	%	Comment
Duraplasty for spinal cord injury[46,47]			
Cerebrospinal fluid leak	4/26	10	Treated successfully with lumbar drain
Wound infection	0/26	0	
Meningitis (septic)	0/26	0	
Pseudomeningocele	5/26	19	All resolved at 6-mo MRI

Patients column spans No./%.

For further discussion of complications see Refs.[46,47]

MRI as lack of CSF around the injured cord.[16] The degree of spinal cord swelling against the dura was associated with increasing AIS grade.

4. *Animal studies.* Reducing ISP by duraplasty or by deletion of the astrocyte water channel aquaporin-4 limiting cord edema, improved outcome in numerous rodent[49–54] and dog[55] SCI studies.

5. *Analogy with TBI.* The dura is nonelastic.[56] It is well-established that the dura restricts brain swelling; decompression for TBI is based on removing bony and dural restrictions, shown to lower mortality in the RESCUEicp RCT.[57] We propose that expansion duraplasty for SCI is also analogous to decompressive craniectomy for TBI.

6. *Syringomyelia.* Another potential benefit of early duraplasty may be to prevent delayed syringomyelia.[58] Syrinx arises when scarring tethers the injured cord to the dura, which causes delayed neurologic deterioration.[59] In rodent SCI models, early duraplasty reduced cord inflammation and scarring, resulting in smaller syrinx formation.[50]

Risks of Expansion Duraplasty

Expansion duraplasty has been reported in 2 series of patients with acute SCIs without serious morbidity or mortality.[46,47] Duraplasty is also performed in Chiari malformation to decompress the cranio-cervical junction. The commonest complications are CSF-related (**Table 2**). The incidence of wound infection is very low (<1%) and easily treated with antibiotics. Septic meningitis is rare.

Reducing Risks of Duraplasty

Several technical nuances may minimize the risks of infection, CSF leak, and pseudomeningocele after duraplasty for SCI:

1. Use running sutures to attach the dural graft to the patient's dura.
2. Avoid fibrin glue that expand and can cause cord compression
3. Use running locking sutures for fascial and skin apposition, providing 2 layers of watertight closure.
4. Place purse-string sutures around probes to tighten the skin against the probe.
5. Apply a waterproof film dressing (eg, Ioban) over the wound for 1 week.
6. Postoperative antibiotic prophylaxis.
7. Place wound drain 'on gravity' for a week.
8. Nurse patients with cervical SCI at 45° upright for a week to reduce cervical CSF pressure.

Randomized Controlled Trials of Expansion Duraplasty in Spinal Cord Injury

A RCT, termed DISCUS (Duraplasty for Injured cervical Spinal Cord with Uncontrolled Swelling) is being planned to test whether expansion duraplasty + bony decompression improves outcome compared with bony decompression alone in patients with AIS A to C cervical SCI. The trial will begin recruiting in 2021 and aims for 222 patients to be randomized 1:1 to each trial arm. The primary outcome is change in motor score at 6 months compared with baseline. The estimated sample size provides 85% power and 5% significance (2-sided) to detect at least 11-point improvement in the change in total limb motor score at 6 months in the intervention arm, allowing 15% patient loss to follow-up. DISCUS includes monitoring of ISP ± MD from the injury site as optional extra.

SUMMARY

Invasive monitoring from the injury site in patients with SCI is feasible. A variety of data can be gathered that may be useful to guide management. A key finding is that after SCI, spinal cord swelling is restricted by the dura resulting in high intraspinal pressure and reduced cord perfusion. A RCT termed DISCUS is being set up to evaluate expansion duraplasty as a novel treatment for SCI. Invasive monitoring from the injury site also will be examined in the DISCUS trial.

CLINICS CARE POINTS

- ISP monitoring at the injury site may be used to guide management after SCI, analogous to ICP monitoring for brain injury.

- Aiming to optimize SCPP makes more sense than targeting blood pressure, because SCPP accounts for ISP.

- The monitoring studies showed that the injured cord swells and is compressed against dura, which causes compartmentalization at the injury site.

- Based on the observation that the swollen, injured cord is compressed against dura, a randomized trial termed DISCUS is being set up to investigate expansion duraplasty as a novel treatment.

ACKNOWLEDGMENTS

The authors thank the Wings for Life Spinal Cord Research Foundation and the Neurosciences Research Foundation for funding our research in spinal cord injury. The authors also thank the UK Efficacy and Mechanism Evaluation (EME) Programme, a Medical Research Council (MRC) and National Institute for Health Research (NIHR) partnership, for funding the DISCUS trial (NIHR130048). The views expressed in this publication are those of the author(s) and not necessarily those of the MRC, NIHR, or the Department of Health and Social Care.

DISCLOSURE

The authors have nothing to disclose.

REFERENCES

1. Hughes JT. The Edwin Smith Surgical Papyrus: an analysis of the first case reports of spinal cord injuries. Paraplegia 1988;26(2):71–82.

2. Marketos SG, Skiadas P. Hippocrates. The father of spine surgery. Spine (Phila Pa 1976) 1999;24(13):1381–7.

3. Markatos K, Korres D, Kaseta MK, et al. Paul of aegina (625-690): his work and his contribution to neurologic surgery: trephinations and laminectomies in the dark ages. World Neurosurg 2018;109:338–41.

4. Donovan WH. Operative and nonoperative management of spinal cord injury. A review. Paraplegia 1994;32(6):375–88.

5. Weiner MF, Silver JR. The origins of the treatment of traumatic spinal injuries. Eur Neurol 2014;72(5–6):363–9.

6. van Middendorp JJ, Hosman AJ, Doi SA. The effects of the timing of spinal surgery after traumatic spinal cord injury: a systematic review and meta-analysis. J Neurotrauma 2013;30(21):1781–94.

7. Fehlings MG, Vaccaro A, Wilson JR, et al. Early versus delayed decompression for traumatic cervical spinal cord injury: results of the Surgical Timing in Acute Spinal Cord Injury Study (STASCIS). PLoS One 2012;7(2):e32037.

8. Piazza M, Schuster J. Timing of surgery after spinal cord injury. Neurosurg Clin N Am 2017;28(1):31–9.

9. Stocchetti N, Carbonara M, Citerio G, et al. Severe traumatic brain injury: targeted management in the intensive care unit. Lancet Neurol 2017;16(6):452–64.

10. Donnelly J, Czosnyka M, Adams H, et al. Twenty-five years of intracranial pressure monitoring after severe traumatic brain injury: a retrospective, single-center analysis. Neurosurgery 2019;85(1):E75–82.

11. Chesnut R, Aguilera S, Buki A, et al. A management algorithm for adult patients with both brain oxygen and intracranial pressure monitoring: the Seattle International Severe Traumatic Brain Injury Consensus Conference (SIBICC). Intensive Care Med 2020;46(5):919–29.

12. Oddo M, Hutchinson PJ. Understanding and monitoring brain injury: the role of cerebral microdialysis. Intensive Care Med 2018;44(11):1945–8.

13. Werndle MC, Saadoun S, Phang I, et al. Monitoring of spinal cord perfusion pressure in acute spinal cord injury: initial findings of the injured spinal cord pressure evaluation study*. Crit Care Med 2014;42(3):646–55.

14. Werndle MC, Saadoun S, Phang I, et al. Measurement of intraspinal pressure after spinal cord injury: technical note from the injured spinal cord pressure evaluation study. Acta Neurochir Suppl 2016;122:323–8.

15. Varsos GV, Werndle MC, Czosnyka ZH, et al. Intraspinal pressure and spinal cord perfusion pressure after spinal cord injury: an observational study. J Neurosurg Spine 2015;23(6):763–71.

16. Saadoun S, Werndle MC, Lopez de Heredia L, et al. The dura causes spinal cord compression after spinal cord injury. Br J Neurosurg 2016;30(5):582–4.

17. Gallagher MJ, Zoumprouli A, Phang I, et al. Markedly deranged injury site metabolism and impaired

functional recovery in acute spinal cord patients with fever. Crit Care Med 2018;46(7):1150–7.

18. Hogg FRA, Gallagher MJ, Kearney S, et al. Acute spinal cord injury: monitoring lumbar cerebrospinal fluid provides limited information about the injury site. J Neurotrauma 2020;37(9):1156–64.

19. Chen S, Gallagher MJ, Hogg F, et al. Visibility graph analysis of intraspinal pressure signal predicts functional outcome in spinal cord injured patients. J Neurotrauma 2018;35(24):2947–56.

20. Chen S, Gallagher MJ, Papadopoulos MC, et al. Non-linear dynamical analysis of intraspinal pressure signal predicts outcome after spinal cord injury. Front Neurol 2018;9:493.

21. Phang I, Zoumprouli A, Saadoun S, et al. Safety profile and probe placement accuracy of intraspinal pressure monitoring for traumatic spinal cord injury: Injured Spinal Cord Pressure Evaluation study. J Neurosurg Spine 2016;25(3):398–405.

22. Squair JW, Belanger LM, Tsang A, et al. Spinal cord perfusion pressure predicts neurologic recovery in acute spinal cord injury. Neurology 2017;89(16):1660–7.

23. Kwon BK, Curt A, Belanger LM, et al. Intrathecal pressure monitoring and cerebrospinal fluid drainage in acute spinal cord injury: a prospective randomized trial. J Neurosurg Spine 2009;10(3):181–93.

24. Saadeh YS, Smith BW, Joseph JR, et al. The impact of blood pressure management after spinal cord injury: a systematic review of the literature. Neurosurg Focus 2017;43(5):E20.

25. Czosnyka M, Czosnyka Z, Smielewski P. Pressure reactivity index: journey through the past 20 years. Acta Neurochir (Wien) 2017;159(11):2063–5.

26. Gallagher MJ, Hogg FRA, Zoumprouli A, et al. Spinal cord blood flow in patients with acute spinal cord injuries. J Neurotrauma 2019;36(6):919–29.

27. Chen S, Smielewski P, Czosnyka M, et al. Continuous monitoring and visualization of optimum spinal cord perfusion pressure in patients with acute cord injury. J Neurotrauma 2017;34(21):2941–9.

28. Phang I, Zoumprouli A, Papadopoulos MC, et al. Microdialysis to optimize cord perfusion and drug delivery in spinal cord injury. Ann Neurol 2016;80(4):522–31.

29. Abrahamsson P, Aberg AM, Johansson G, et al. Detection of myocardial ischaemia using surface microdialysis on the beating heart. Clin Physiol Funct Imaging 2011;31(3):175–81.

30. Abrahamsson P, Aberg AM, Winso O, et al. Surface microdialysis sampling: a new approach described in a liver ischaemia model. Clin Physiol Funct Imaging 2012;32(2):99–105.

31. Akesson O, Falkenback D, Johansson G, et al. Surface microdialysis detects ischemia after esophageal resection-an experimental animal study. J Surg Res 2020;245:537–43.

32. Akesson O, Abrahamsson P, Johansson G, et al. Surface microdialysis on small bowel serosa in monitoring of ischemia. J Surg Res 2016;204(1):39–46.

33. Chen S, Phang I, Zoumprouli A, et al. Metabolic profile of injured human spinal cord determined using surface microdialysis. J Neurochem 2016;139(5):700–5.

34. Gallagher MJ, Hogg FRA, Kearney S, et al. Effects of local hypothermia-rewarming on physiology, metabolism and inflammation of acutely injured human spinal cord. Sci Rep 2020;10(1):8125–y.

35. Clifton GL, Valadka A, Zygun D, et al. Very early hypothermia induction in patients with severe brain injury (the National Acute Brain Injury Study: Hypothermia II): a randomised trial. Lancet Neurol 2011;10(2):131–9.

36. Adelson PD, Wisniewski SR, Beca J, et al. Comparison of hypothermia and normothermia after severe traumatic brain injury in children (Cool Kids): a phase 3, randomised controlled trial. Lancet Neurol 2013;12(6):546–53.

37. Andrews PJ, Sinclair HL, Rodriguez A, et al. Hypothermia for intracranial hypertension after traumatic brain injury. N Engl J Med 2015;373(25):2403–12.

38. Bracken MB, Shepard MJ, Collins WF, et al. A randomized, controlled trial of methylprednisolone or naloxone in the treatment of acute spinal-cord injury. Results of the Second National Acute Spinal Cord Injury Study. N Engl J Med 1990;322(20):1405–11.

39. Saadoun S, Chen S, Papadopoulos MC. Intraspinal pressure and spinal cord perfusion pressure predict neurological outcome after traumatic spinal cord injury. J Neurol Neurosurg Psychiatry 2017;88(5):452–3.

40. Saadoun S, Papadopoulos MC. Spinal cord injury: is monitoring from the injury site the future? Crit Care 2016;20(1):308–13.

41. Hennekens CH, Ds D. Statistical association and causation: contributions of different types of evidence. JAMA 2011;305(11):1134–5.

42. Seth AK, Barnett L. Granger causality analysis in neuroscience and neuroimaging. J Neurosci 2015;35(8):3293–7.

43. Hogg FRA, Kearney S, Zoumprouli A, et al. Acute spinal cord injury: correlations and causal relations between intraspinal pressure, spinal cord perfusion pressure, lactate-to-pyruvate ratio, and limb power. Neurocrit Care 2020;34(1):121–9.

44. Inoue T, Manley GT, Patel N, et al. Medical and surgical management after spinal cord injury: vasopressor usage, early surgerys, and complications. J Neurotrauma 2014;31(3):284–91.

45. Readdy WJ, Whetstone WD, Ferguson AR, et al. Complications and outcomes of vasopressor usage in acute traumatic central cord syndrome. J Neurosurg Spine 2015;23(5):574–80.

46. Phang I, Werndle MC, Saadoun S, et al. Expansion duraplasty improves intraspinal pressure, spinal cord perfusion pressure, and vascular pressure reactivity index in patients with traumatic spinal cord injury: injured spinal cord pressure evaluation study. J Neurotrauma 2015;32(12):865–74.

47. Zhu F, Yao S, Ren Z, et al. Early durotomy with duraplasty for severe adult spinal cord injury without radiographic abnormality: a novel concept and method of surgical decompression. Eur Spine J 2019;28(10):2275–82.

48. Hogg FRA, Gallagher MJ, Chen S, et al. Predictors of intraspinal pressure and optimal cord perfusion pressure after traumatic spinal cord injury. Neurocrit Care 2019;30(2):421–8.

49. Zhang J, Wang H, Zhang C, et al. Intrathecal decompression versus epidural decompression in the treatment of severe spinal cord injury in rat model: a randomized, controlled preclinical research. J Orthop Surg Res 2016;11:34–y.

50. Iannotti C, Zhang YP, Shields LB, et al. Dural repair reduces connective tissue scar invasion and cystic cavity formation after acute spinal cord laceration injury in adult rats. J Neurotrauma 2006;23(6):853–65.

51. Saadoun S, Bell BA, Verkman AS, et al. Greatly improved neurological outcome after spinal cord compression injury in AQP4-deficient mice. Brain 2008;131(Pt 4):1087–98.

52. Fernandez E, Pallini R. Connective tissue scarring in experimental spinal cord lesions: significance of dural continuity and role of epidural tissues. Acta Neurochir (Wien) 1985;76(3–4):145–8.

53. Jalan D, Saini N, Zaidi M, et al. Effects of early surgical decompression on functional and histological outcomes after severe experimental thoracic spinal cord injury. J Neurosurg Spine 2017;26(1):62–75.

54. Smith JS, Anderson R, Pham T, et al. Role of early surgical decompression of the intradural space after cervical spinal cord injury in an animal model. J Bone Joint Surg Am 2010;92(5):1206–14.

55. Jeffery ND, Mankin JM, Ito D, et al. Extended durotomy to treat severe spinal cord injury after acute thoracolumbar disc herniation in dogs. Vet Surg 2020;49(5):884–93.

56. Wilcox RK, Bilston LE, Barton DC, et al. Mathematical model for the viscoelastic properties of dura mater. J Orthop Sci 2003;8(3):432–4.

57. Hutchinson PJ, Kolias AG, Timofeev IS, et al. Trial of decompressive craniectomy for traumatic intracranial hypertension. N Engl J Med 2016;375(12):1119–30.

58. Kleindienst A, Laut FM, Roeckelein V, et al. Treatment of posttraumatic syringomyelia: evidence from a systematic review. Acta Neurochir (Wien) 2020;162(10):2541–56.

59. Falci SP, Indeck C, Lammertse DP. Posttraumatic spinal cord tethering and syringomyelia: surgical treatment and long-term outcome. J Neurosurg Spine 2009;11(4):445–60.

Hypothermia for Acute Spinal Cord Injury

Aditya Vedantam, MD, Allan D. Levi, MD, PhD*

KEYWORDS

• Hypothermia • Spinal cord injury • Neuroprotection • Cooling catheter • Trauma

KEY POINTS

- Systemic hypothermia is a proven neuroprotective strategy to limit secondary injury in animal models of acute spinal cord injury.
- Modest hypothermia (32–34 °C) has been shown to provide effective neuroprotection with fewer adverse effects as compared with profound hypothermia (<28 °C).
- Endovascular cooling allows for rapid induction of systemic hypothermia and tight control of body temperature.
- The University of Miami is leading a multicenter randomized controlled trial to evaluate the efficacy of modest therapeutic hypothermia for acute cervical spinal cord injury.

INTRODUCTION

Spinal cord injury (SCI) can cause devastating motor, sensory, and autonomic deficits. The treatment of acute SCI is aimed at preventing secondary injury and promoting neural repair. Currently, there are no proven therapeutic interventions for acute SCI, although a number of candidate drugs and therapies are being evaluated. Systemic hypothermia, a proven neuroprotective strategy,[1] is a promising therapeutic intervention to limit secondary injury after acute SCI.

Therapeutic hypothermia has been extensively studied in both the preclinical and clinical settings for a variety of conditions.[2] Clinical trials have evaluated the use of hypothermia for traumatic brain injury,[3] stroke,[4] and neuroprotection after out-of-hospital cardiac arrest,[5,6] perinatal hypoxia,[7] and ischemic damage post aortic aneurysm repair.[8] These studies provide robust data for the clinical feasibility and safety of systemic hypothermia after acute central nervous system injury. Data from our center on systemic hypothermia for acute SCI has provided further encouraging data for the neuroprotective effect of systemic hypothermia.[9–11]

In the present article, we describe the history of hypothermia, its mechanism of neuroprotection, and results from animal and human studies, as well as the current status of trials for hypothermia in acute SCI.

HISTORY OF HYPOTHERMIA IN HUMANS

Clinical experience with therapeutic hypothermia dates back to the 1950s when hypothermia was induced for patients after cardiac arrest.[12] However, these early studies did not show consistent benefit for the use of therapeutic hypothermia, and many aspects of technique were not well defined. Profound hypothermia, which was used in most of these studies, produced considerable side effects, including coagulopathy, infections, and arrhythmias.[13] Due to these issues, as well as promising preliminary results from treating SCI with pharmacologic agents, interest in the use of therapeutic hypothermia waned for a few decades. In the 1990s, mild hypothermia emerged as a treatment for patients undergoing surgical clipping of cerebral aneurysms,[14] traumatic brain injury,[15] and cardiac arrest.[16] In 2002, 2 clinical trials showed that therapeutic mild hypothermia led

Department of Neurological Surgery, University of Miami MILLER School of Medicine, Lois Pope Life Center, 1095 Northwest 14th Terrace, Suite 2-24, Miami, FL 33136, USA
* Corresponding author.
E-mail address: ALevi@med.miami.edu

Neurosurg Clin N Am 32 (2021) 377–387
https://doi.org/10.1016/j.nec.2021.03.009
1042-3680/21/© 2021 Elsevier Inc. All rights reserved.

to increased survival and superior neurologic outcomes for patients with out-of-hospital cardiac arrest.[5,6] These data have led to renewed interest in the neuroprotective effects of therapeutic hypothermia.

The history of hypothermia in patients with SCI began in the 1960s with local cooling using cold saline after decompressive surgery. In some of the early studies, the spinal cord was directly exposed with durotomy and cooled with direct application of ice cold saline.[17,18] Although the intervention led to functional improvement in many of these patients, it was difficult to tease out the independent benefit of hypothermia because of the retrospective nature of the reports. Some of these patients may have improved due to decompressive surgery, medical therapy or even selection bias. Additional evidence for the neuroprotective effect of hypothermia came from studies that used hypothermia during thoracoabdominal aortic aneurysm repair.[8,19] In these studies, systemic hypothermia was associated with lower rates of ischemic SCI while crossclamping the aorta. Put together, these data suggest that there is clinical evidence for neuroprotection from hypothermia for SCI.

Definitions of Hypothermia and Rewarming

The temperatures that define different hypothermia protocols are variable. In general, moderate hypothermia is defined as target temperatures of 28 to 32 °C, whereas mild hypothermia ranges from 33 to 36 °C.[20] Data from animal studies suggest that an intermediate temperature between mild and moderate provides effective neuroprotection[21,22] and therefore, the term "modest hypothermia" (32–34 °C) is used to define the target temperature in our hypothermia protocol for acute SCI.[9]

Early induction of hypothermia after injury, shorter time to target temperature (0.5–2.0 °C per hour), prolonged duration of hypothermia (24–48 hours) and slow rewarming (0.1 °C per hour) are critical for an effective hypothermia protocol for SCI. These clinical criteria are based on animal experiments as well as early clinical experience with therapeutic hypothermia. Rapid rewarming can reverse the neuroprotective effects of hypothermia and is associated with significant morbidity.[23] At the cellular level, rapid rewarming can cause the release of proinflammatory cytokines, worsening edema due to rebound vasodilation, and more severe neural injury.[24,25] For these reasons, it has become standard practice to increase body temperature gradually in the order of 0.1 °C per hour after termination of the hypothermia protocol.[26]

MECHANISMS OF ACTION OF HYPOTHERMIA FOR NEUROPROTECTION

Hypothermia affects various physiologic and biochemical processes at the cellular level. The effect on these processes can play a role in preventing secondary injury after SCI.[27] Hypothermia lowers cellular metabolic activity and energy consumption within tissues.[28] The reduced metabolic rate provides protection against energy depletion during brief periods of ischemia,[29,30] thereby protecting the tissues that have sustained stress or injury. Animal studies have also demonstrated that hypothermia can attenuate glutamate excitotoxicity in the central nervous system by modulating the AMPA and NMDA glutamate receptors.[31,32]

One of the most effective ways by which hypothermia provides neuroprotection is by reducing inflammation and oxidative stress. Hypothermia can alter matrix metalloproteinases and attenuate breakdown of the blood brain barrier,[33] thereby reducing the extravasation of inflammatory cells.[21] Hypothermia inhibits microglial activation[34] as well as release of proinflammatory cytokines[35] and reactive oxygen species[36] after central nervous system injury. In addition to reducing inflammation and edema, hypothermia can decrease the rate of apoptotic neuronal cell death in SCI.[37]

The effect of hypothermia on physiologic processes is dependent on the target temperature. Severe hypothermia works primarily by reducing oxygen consumption, whereas mild and moderate hypothermia provide neuroprotection by many different mechanisms, as described previously.[27]

ANIMAL EVIDENCE FOR HYPOTHERMIA AFTER SPINAL CORD INJURY
Regional Hypothermia

Therapeutic benefits of regional and systemic hypothermia have been evaluated using animal models of SCI.[38] Various techniques have been used to produce local intradural or epidural cooling of the spinal cord after experimental SCI. The results of regional hypothermia in animal SCI models have not been consistently positive. Although many studies showed that local cooling improved functional and motor outcomes after experimental SCI, other studies reported negative results.[39] Ha and Kim[34] maintained an epidural temperature of 30 °C for 48 hours after thoracic SCI and found that hindlimb motor function and strength improved significantly in the treatment group. Casas and colleagues[40] found no significant benefit of epidural cooling (24–35 °C) in terms of locomotor outcome, or tissue preservation after moderate thoracic spinal cord contusions in rats. Morochovic and colleagues[41] found that local transcutaneous cooling (~28.5 °C) produced tissue preservation, but this did not result in functional improvement. A few other factors that appear to impact outcomes after treatment of experimental SCI with local cooling include the type of animal SCI model, the duration of local hypothermia, and how soon after the injury hypothermia is initiated. Dimar and colleagues[42] showed that profound local hypothermia (19 °C) was effective in a rat model of spinal cord compression using an epidural spacer but not after a weight-drop spinal cord contusion. In one study, local epidural cooling (28 °C for 48 hours) and systemic hypothermia (32 °C for 48 hours) were compared using a rat spinal cord contusion model. The investigators found that although there were no significant differences in functional outcomes, systemic hypothermia was superior to local epidural cooling with regard to markers of apoptosis within the injured tissue.[43]

Systemic Hypothermia

Moderate systemic hypothermia has been shown to improve outcomes in animal SCI models. A meta-analysis of preclinical studies showed a predictable improvement in behavioral outcomes for animals treated with systemic hypothermia after acute SCI.[38] Maybhate and colleagues[44] showed that moderate systemic hypothermia (32 °C for 2 hours, initiated at 2 hours postinjury) produced improvements in somatosensory evoked potentials and motor function, as well as contributed to tissue preservation in a rat SCI contusion model. The improvements in motor function were sustained at 28 days after injury. Batchelor and colleagues[45] attempted to replicate the clinical scenario of a patient undergoing delayed decompressive surgery after acute SCI. The investigators used systemic hypothermia as a bridge between the time from injury and spinal cord decompression. Systemic hypothermia (33 °C) was initiated 30 minutes after contusive injury and maintained for 7.5 hours until the spinal cord compression was relieved. The investigators showed that the use of moderate systemic hypothermia was associated with improved locomotor function as well as histologic evidence of white and gray matter preservation in the spinal cord. Several studies have provided additional data on neuroprotective effects of systemic hypothermia at the cellular level and in terms of functional outcomes.[37,46–51] Hypothermia has been shown to have a beneficial effect on recovery from SCI, when combined with other neuroprotective therapies.[52,53] Data from animal studies also indicate that early initiation of hypothermia,[49] as well as maintenance of moderate systemic hypothermia for prolonged duration[46] is necessary for effective neuroprotection after SCI.

HUMAN EVIDENCE FOR HYPOTHERMIA AFTER SPINAL CORD INJURY
Regional Hypothermia

As a historical note, the surgical treatment of SCI in 1960s and 1970s involved laminectomy and durotomy. After the durotomy, the injured spinal cord was continuously irrigated with ice cold saline (1–3 °C) to create profound local hypothermia.[17,18] Only a few studies with small sample sizes were performed and the results could not definitively confirm the independent effect of hypothermia on outcomes.[17,54–56] In one study, localized spinal cord cooling using ice cold irrigation was initiated within 3 hours in 4 patients with acute SCI as well as chronic SCI. Only 1 of the patients with acute SCI showed improvement in motor function.[54] Subsequently, other studies showed mild improvement in motor function in patients with acute SCI with local hypothermia.[17,55,56] Localized cooling was performed after decompressive laminectomy, and using iced saline solutions to irrigate the spinal cord. Many of these patients also received steroids as part of treatment for acute SCI.[18] Hansebout and Hansebout[57] recently described one of the largest series of acute SCI treated with local hypothermia. The investigators used a custom local epidural cooling device to keep the dural temperature at 6 °C for up to 4 hours. All 20 patients were American Spinal Injury Association (ASIA) Impairment Scale (AIS) A (cervical or thoracic SCI) at admission and underwent decompressive surgery and/or fusion within 8 hours of injury. The investigators found improvement in at least 1 AIS grade in 80% of patients at a mean follow-up approaching 5 years. Although there is evidence for neurologic improvement patients treated with local hypothermia, the quality of evidence from these studies is low. The presence of significant confounders, such as decompressive surgery with or without durotomy, and use of corticosteroids make it difficult to discern the independent benefit of local hypothermia. In one experimental primate SCI study, the investigators compared neurologic outcome between normothermic and hypothermic local perfusion of the spinal cord after durotomy. Neurologic improvement was superior in the group that received normothermic perfusion, suggesting that neuroprotection may not be solely related to hypothermic fluid, but also the removal of noxious cytokines from the intrathecal space.[58]

Early induction of local cooling and maintenance of regional hypothermia for a prolonged duration after acute SCI has proven difficult because of the need for an open durotomy, indwelling subdural catheters, and extended sedation. Technical barriers remain difficult to overcome. Accordingly, local cooling is not currently under widespread investigation.

Systemic Hypothermia in Human Spinal Cord Injury

Techniques
Surface cooling The application of ice packs, cooling blankets or cooling pads to the skin can produce systemic hypothermia by surface cooling.[1] Cooling blankets can produce hypothermia by circulating cold air or water. These methods can decrease the body temperature without the need for any invasive procedures, and therefore can be easily applied, even at the trauma scene. Newer systems, such as cooling blankets (Arctic Sun [Medivance, Louisville, CO], **Fig. 1**) are able to produce systemic hypothermia faster than ice packs. Some of the challenges with surface cooling include the slow rate (4–8 hours) of inducing mild hypothermia,[59] the physiologic shivering response, and the difficulty in achieving the target temperature in obese patients. In addition, maintenance of the target temperature can be difficult

with surface cooling, as this system does not allow for tight control of body temperature (**Fig. 2**).[60]

Cold intravenous infusion cooling Cold intravenous fluids such as ice cold saline have been used as an effective means to reduce body temperature. These can be administered through peripheral intravenous lines and therefore, can be started in the field soon after the injury to rapidly decrease body temperature. Ice cold intravenous fluids have been used for rapid induction of hypothermia after cardiac arrest.[61,62] Given the volume of intravenous fluids required to maintain hypothermia, these cannot be administered for prolonged periods. Therefore, surface cooling or endovascular cooling is needed to further maintain the systemic hypothermia.

Endovascular cooling Intravascular cooling catheters are superior to surface cooling techniques to induce and maintain systemic hypothermia.[63] Commercially available cooling catheters include Quattro, Icy and Cool Line (Zoll, Chelmsford, MA), and these are connected to an external machine (Thermogard XP [Zoll, Chelmsford, MA], **Fig. 3**) that controls the temperature of the cooling balloons. The catheter is inserted via a percutaneous technique and the tip of the catheter is placed in the inferior vena cava. These catheters can also be inserted into the subclavian or internal

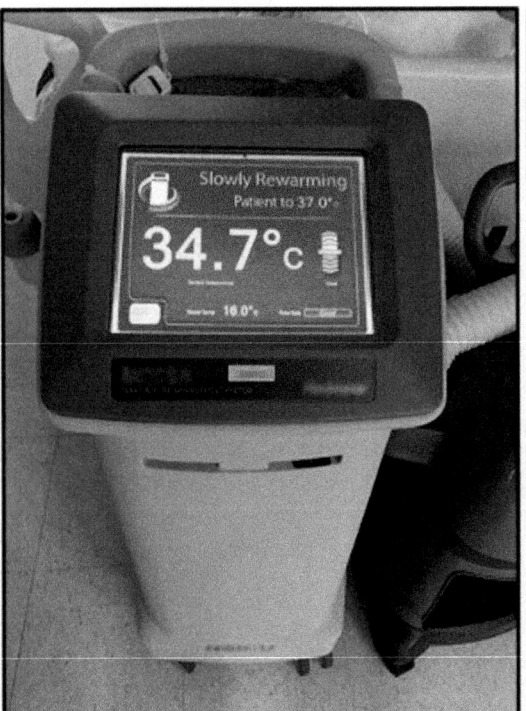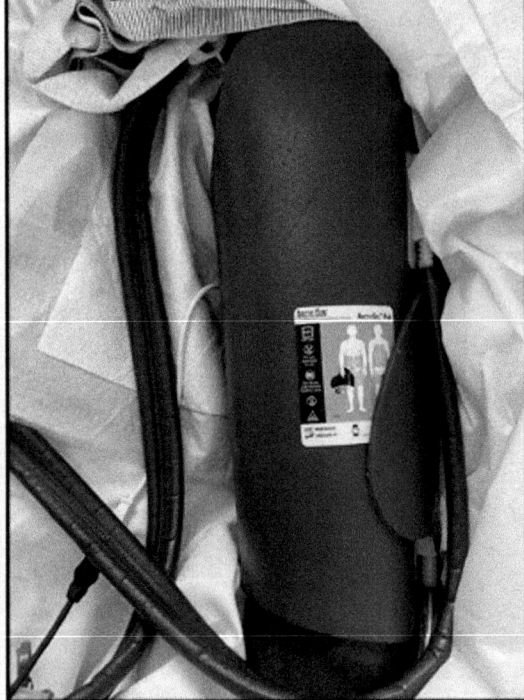

Fig. 1. Surface cooling gel pads and temperature management system.

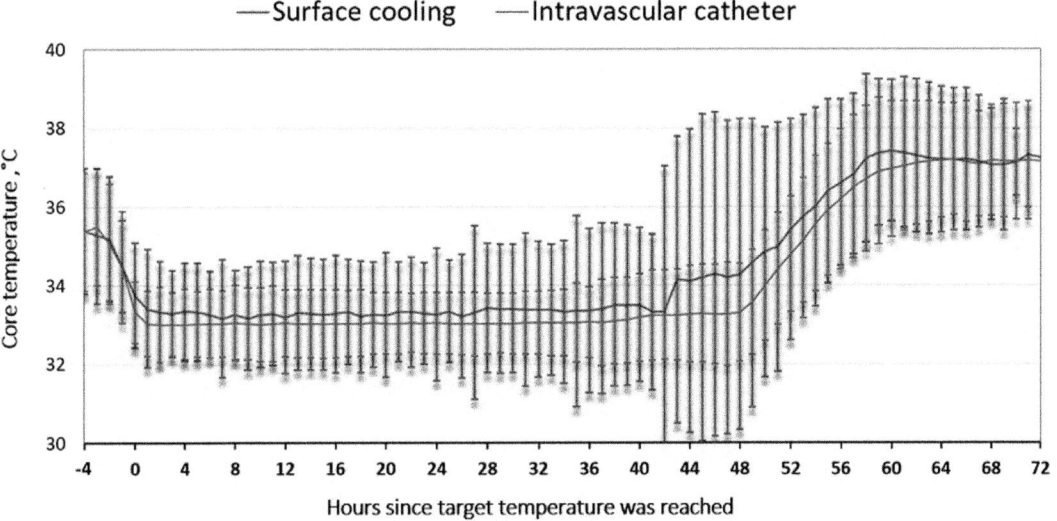

— Surface cooling   — Intravascular catheter

Fig. 2. Mean (±SD) temperature graph showing more rapid achievement of target temperature and tighter control of target in patients with out-of-hospital cardiac arrest. (Published under the terms of the Creative Commons Attribution 4.0 from De Fazio C et al. Intravascular versus surface cooling for targeted temperature management after out-of-hospital cardiac arrest: an analysis of the TTH48 trial. *Crit Care.* 2019;23(1):61.)

jugular vein. Saline is cooled in the external machine to 4 to 5 °C and pushed into the cooling balloons that are mounted on the catheter. The blood that comes into contact with the catheter is cooled and a temperature probe on the catheter allows for closed loop monitoring of temperature. The external machine regulates the temperature of the saline to maintain the target temperature specified by the physician. The catheter has additional ports for medications and infusions. The rate of

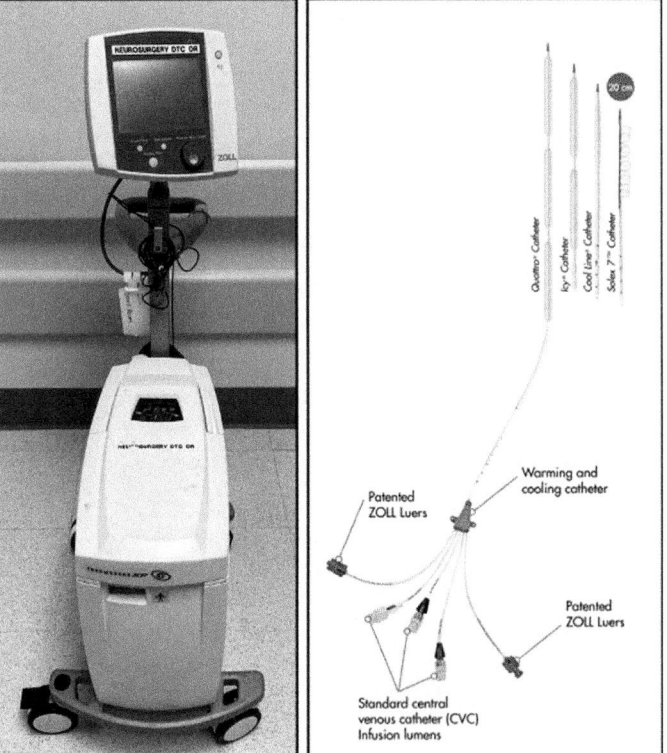

Fig. 3. Central venous cooling catheter (Icy Catheter) and temperature management system. (*Courtesy of* Zoll Medical Corp, Chelmsford, MA.)

cooling is reported to be 2 to 4 °C per hour, and so these systems can rapidly induce systemic hypothermia.[13,63] Unlike cold intravenous infusions, these systems do not add any additional intravascular volume.

Clinical studies

The University of Miami has published several articles including an initial techniques paper,[9] the 1-year outcomes on our first 14 patients,[10] followed by the largest series of patients with acute SCI treated with modest systemic hypothermia.[11] The initial outcomes paper in adult patients with acute traumatic cervical SCI (ASIA A) were recruited between 2006 and 2008, and underwent systemic hypothermia by endovascular cooling.[9] The catheter was inserted via percutaneous puncture of the femoral vein and the tip was positioned in the inferior vena cava. The target temperature was 33 °C and maintained for 48 hours. The patients were then rewarmed at 0.1 °C/hour to 37 °C (**Fig. 4**). Other neuroprotective strategies included maintaining a mean arterial pressure greater than 90 mm Hg at all times. This study highlighted the feasibility of this technique in the clinical setting for acute SCI, as well as some of the areas for improvement in future studies. Some of the salient features of this study include the fact that average time to initiation of hypothermia was 6.15 ± 0.7 hours, after excluding 2 outliers. The average time from initiation of hypothermia to reaching the target temperature was 2.75 ± 0.75 hours. Importantly, all patients underwent surgical intervention, and this was performed during the cooling phase or at the target temperature. Given the importance of early surgical decompression for acute SCI, this study highlighted the safety of operating on hypothermic patients with acute SCI. One of the important physiologic results of this study was the linear association between bradycardia and lower body temperature. Despite the safety and feasibility of the hypothermia protocol, we identified that the time between SCI and initiation of hypothermia could be improved by implementing a more rapid hypothermia induction protocol. We feel it might be possible to initiate hypothermia at the trauma scene by administering cold intravenous fluids, augmented by the insertion of magnetic resonance-compatible cooling catheters in the emergency room.

We subsequently published 1-year follow-up data from our initial study, further describing the neurologic outcomes for 14 patients with AIS A cervical SCI.[10] A matched cohort of patients with AIS A cervical SCI, who did not undergo systemic hypothermia, was used for comparison. Six (42.8%) of the 14 patients treated with hypothermia had an improved AIS grade at follow-up (mean 50.2 weeks). Three patients improved to AIS B, 2 patients improved to AIS C, and 1 patient improved to AIS D at final follow-up. In the control group, improvement was seen in 3 (21.4%) of 14 patients, with 1 patient each converting to AIS B, C, and D. Complications during the hospital stay were not significantly different between the 2 groups, further emphasizing the safety of modest systemic hypothermia in acute cervical SCI. Interest in systemic hypothermia for SCI increased following the case report of a professional football

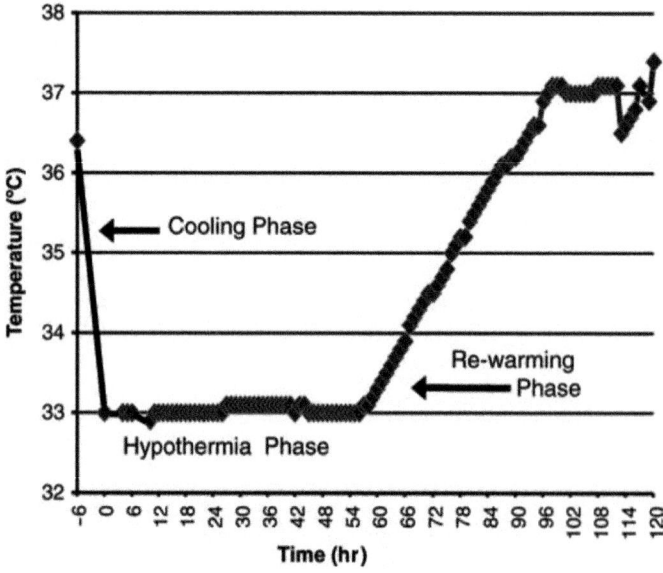

Fig. 4. Temperature curve for a patient undergoing modest hypothermia after acute SCI showing 3 phases of temperature control. (Figure is reproduced from Levi AD et al. Clinical application of modest hypothermia after spinal cord injury. *J Neurotrauma*. 2009;26(3):407-415; with permission from Mary Ann Liebert, Inc.)

player who underwent modest systemic hypothermia after sustaining a AIS A acute cervical SCI on the field.[64] The patient was treated with intravenous steroids, early surgery, and modest systemic hypothermia (surface and endovascular cooling). The patient had a remarkable recovery to AIS D at early follow-up, and continued to improve at his 9-year follow-up.[65]

In our next publication, we published our larger experience of 35 patients with acute cervical SCI who underwent modest systemic hypothermia.[11] Twenty-one patients in this study were prospectively studied. Of the 35 patients, 4 patients converted from AIS A to AIS B within 24 hours of injury. Of the 31 patients who were AIS A at 24 hours after injury, improvement by at least 1 AIS grade was noted in 11 patients (35.5%). Early surgical decompression was performed in most patients (83%). These data provide additional evidence for the safety of modest systemic hypothermia for acute SCI. The rate of neurologic improvement, measured by the AIS grade, also compared favorably with prior data on AIS conversion after SCI.[66] The results of our experience with systemic hypothermia for acute cervical SCI also provided the impetus for a randomized trial.

In May 2017, our team initiated a multicenter randomized controlled trial (NCT02991690) to evaluate the efficacy of modest therapeutic hypothermia for acute cervical SCI. This study is recruiting, with a target enrollment of 120 patients. Inclusion and exclusion criteria are shown in **Table 1**.

Endovascular cooling is initiated within 24 hours postinjury to maintain modest hypothermia (33 °C) for 48 hours. Primary outcome measures are neurologic improvement at 12 months based on the AIS grade and ASIA motor score. Secondary outcome measures are improvement in the Functional Independence Measure and Spinal Cord Independence Measure at 12 months. To date, the study has recruited 36 patients with acute cervical SCI across 6 institutions in the United States.

COMPLICATIONS OF THERAPEUTIC HYPOTHERMIA AND REWARMING

Early reports focused on the side effects and complications of deep systemic hypothermia. These side effects are less pronounced with the use of mild and modest systemic hypothermia. Deep hypothermia can cause profound decreases in myocardial contractility as well as increased risk of arrhythmias. It can also trigger atrial fibrillation, which can progress to ventricular tachycardia and ventricular fibrillation with further decreases in temperature. Prolonged PR and QT intervals and widened QRS complexes are the most common electrocardiographic changes. All levels of hypothermia produce bradycardia that may occasionally need to be treated with medications or pacing.[67]

Hypothermia can increase the risk of coagulopathy. Even mild hypothermia causes platelet dysfunction and thrombocytopenia. Significant

Table 1
Inclusion and exclusion criteria for randomized clinical trial of systemic hypothermia in acute cervical spinal cord injury (NCT02991690, available at clinicaltrials.gov)

Inclusion Criteria	Exclusion Criteria
18–70 y of age	Age > 70 y
American Spinal Injury Association Impairment Scale (AIS) Grade A–C	AIS Grade D
Glasgow Coma Scale ≥14	Hyperthermia on admission (>38.5°C)
Able to start hypothermia treatment within 24 h of injury	Severe systemic injury
Nonpenetrating injury	Severe bleeding
Patients urgently taken to the operating room for surgical reduction also may be included	Pregnancy
	Coagulopathy
	Thrombocytopenia
	Known prior severe cardiac history
	Blood dyscrasia
	Pancreatitis
	Reynaud syndrome
	Cord transection

coagulopathy is often seen only in deep hypothermia. In our experience, there were no challenges obtaining hemostasis or complications related to bleeding for patients with SCI undergoing spinal surgery during modest systemic hypothermia.[9] Because hypothermia produces a considerable anti-inflammatory effect, there is an increased risk of infection in patients undergoing systemic hypothermia. Many physiologic responses to infection are suppressed under hypothermia; hence, the threshold to investigate and treat suspected infection should be low.[68] However, we found no significantly increased rate of infections in patients with acute SCI treated with modest hypothermia, when compared with patients with acute SCI not undergoing hypothermia.[10]

Systemic hypothermia induces cutaneous vasoconstriction and shivering. Cutaneous vasoconstriction increases the risk of poor wound healing and development of pressure sores. Shivering is a physiologic heat-generating response of the body to hypothermia. Shivering increases the metabolic rate and oxygen consumption, as well as raises the body temperature.[13] Some drugs that are effective in counteracting shivering include meperidine and magnesium. Adequate sedation and analgesia can also prevent the shivering response. Hypothermia increases the excretion of magnesium, phosphorous, and potassium, and thereby affects serum electrolyte concentrations. Other side effects include gastroparesis, constipation, and impaired drug clearance. The use of indwelling endovascular cooling catheters does carry the risk of deep vein thrombosis.[69,70] This risk is compounded by immobility due to SCI. The risk can be decreased by the use of sequential compression devices, early initiation of prophylactic anticoagulation, and early removal of the catheter once hypothermia is terminated.

Controlling the rate of rewarming is essential to prevent complications. Rapid rewarming can cause hyperkalemia due to shifts into the extracellular compartment, and can increase insulin sensitivity producing hypoglycemia. It can also initiate an inflammatory cascade and reverse the neuroprotective effect of hypothermia.[7]

SUMMARY

Preclinical and clinical evidence for neuroprotection using systemic hypothermia is robust. The mechanisms of action have been well studied, and the multiple pathophysiological processes affected by hypothermia make it an attractive treatment modality for neuroprotection. Improvements in techniques to induce systemic hypothermia and the relative safety of modest hypothermia

have helped translate this therapy for human use. Our experience with systemic hypothermia for acute SCI provides data on its potential role for neuroprotection in human SCI. The results of the ongoing multicenter randomized trial may provide level I evidence, for the first time, for the role of systemic hypothermia in acute SCI.

CLINICS CARE POINTS

- Modest hypothermia (32–34 °C) is safe and feasible early after acute SCI.
- Early induction of hypothermia, short time to target temperature (<2 hours), maintenance of hypothermia for 48 hours, and slow rewarming (0.1 °C per hour) are critical for an effective hypothermia protocol.
- Endovascular cooling catheters, which are MRI compatible, can be inserted in the emergency room to rapidly induce hypothermia after acute SCI, and this can be supplemented with cooling blankets.
- Surgical interventions can be performed during the cooling phase or at the target temperature without significantly increased risks.
- Bradycardia is common in patients treated with systemic hypothermia, and this may need treatment with medications or pacing.

DISCLOSURE

The authors have nothing to disclose. The authors report no commercial or financial conflicts of interest.

REFERENCES

1. Alzaga AG, Cerdan M, Varon J. Therapeutic hypothermia. Resuscitation 2006;70(3):369–80.
2. Bohl MA, Martirosyan NL, Killeen ZW, et al. The history of therapeutic hypothermia and its use in neurosurgery. J Neurosurg 2018;1–15.
3. Andrews PJ, Sinclair HL, Rodriguez A, et al. Hypothermia for intracranial hypertension after traumatic brain injury. N Engl J Med 2015;373:2403–12.
4. Schwab S, Schwarz S, Spranger M, et al. Moderate hypothermia in the treatment of patients with severe middle cerebral artery infarction. Stroke 1998; 29(12):2461–6.
5. Bernard SA, Gray TW, Buist MD, et al. Treatment of comatose survivors of out-of-hospital cardiac arrest

with induced hypothermia. N Engl J Med 2002; 346(8):557–63.

6. Hypothermia after Cardiac Arrest Study Group. Mild therapeutic hypothermia to improve the neurologic outcome after cardiac arrest. N Engl J Med 2002; 346(8):549–56.

7. Jacobs SE, Berg M, Hunt R, et al. Cooling for newborns with hypoxic ischaemic encephalopathy. Cochrane Database Syst Rev 2013;(1):CD003311.

8. Rokkas CK, Kouchoukos NT. Profound hypothermia for spinal cord protection in operations on the descending thoracic and thoracoabdominal aorta. Semin Thorac Cardiovasc Surg 1998;10(1):57–60.

9. Levi AD, Green BA, Wang MY, et al. Clinical application of modest hypothermia after spinal cord injury. J Neurotrauma 2009;26(3):407–15.

10. Levi AD, Casella G, Green BA, et al. Clinical outcomes using modest intravascular hypothermia after acute cervical spinal cord injury. Neurosurgery 2010;66(4):670–7.

11. Dididze M, Green BA, Dietrich WD, et al. Systemic hypothermia in acute cervical spinal cord injury: a case-controlled study. Spinal Cord 2013;51(5): 395–400.

12. Williams GR, Spencer FC. The clinical use of hypothermia following cardiac arrest. Ann Surg 1958; 148(3):462–8.

13. Polderman KH. Application of therapeutic hypothermia in the ICU: opportunities and pitfalls of a promising treatment modality. Part 1: Indications and evidence. Intensive Care Med 2004;30(4):556–75.

14. Lawton MT, Raudzens PA, Zabramski JM, et al. Hypothermic circulatory arrest in neurovascular surgery: evolving indications and predictors of patient outcome. Neurosurgery 1998;43(1):10–20 [discussion 20-21].

15. Shiozaki T, Sugimoto H, Taneda M, et al. Effect of mild hypothermia on uncontrollable intracranial hypertension after severe head injury. J Neurosurg 1993;79(3):363–8.

16. Yanagawa Y, Ishihara S, Norio H, et al. Preliminary clinical outcome study of mild resuscitative hypothermia after out-of-hospital cardiopulmonary arrest. Resuscitation 1998;39(1–2):61–6.

17. Demian YK, White RJ, Yashon D, et al. Anaesthesia for laminectomy and localized cord cooling in acute cervical spine injury. Report of three cases. Br J Anaesth 1971;43(10):973–9.

18. Bricolo A, Ore GD, Da Pian R, et al. Local cooling in spinal cord injury. Surg Neurol 1976;6(2):101–6.

19. Kouchoukos NT. Hypothermic circulatory arrest and hypothermic perfusion for extensive disease of the thoracic and thoracoabdominal aorta. Jpn J Thorac Cardiovasc Surg 1999;47(1):1–5.

20. Inamasu J, Ichikizaki K. Mild hypothermia in neurologic emergency: an update. Ann Emerg Med 2002;40(2):220–30.

21. Chatzipanteli K, Yanagawa Y, Marcillo AE, et al. Posttraumatic hypothermia reduces polymorphonuclear leukocyte accumulation following spinal cord injury in rats. J Neurotrauma 2000;17(4):321–32.

22. Busto R, Dietrich WD, Globus MY, et al. Small differences in intraischemic brain temperature critically determine the extent of ischemic neuronal injury. J Cereb Blood Flow Metab 1987;7(6):729–38.

23. Povlishock JT, Wei EP. Posthypothermic rewarming considerations following traumatic brain injury. J Neurotrauma 2009;26(3):333–40.

24. Berger C, Xia F, Köhrmann M, et al. Hypothermia in acute stroke–slow versus fast rewarming an experimental study in rats. Exp Neurol 2007;204(1):131–7.

25. Zhu S-Z, Gu Y, Wu Z, et al. Hypothermia followed by rapid rewarming exacerbates ischemia-induced brain injury and augments inflammatory response in rats. Biochem Biophys Res Commun 2016; 474(1):175–81.

26. Ahmad FU, Wang MY, Levi AD. Hypothermia for acute spinal cord injury–a review. World Neurosurg 2014;82(1–2):207–14.

27. Dietrich WD, Atkins CM, Bramlett HM. Protection in animal models of brain and spinal cord injury with mild to moderate hypothermia. J Neurotrauma 2009;26(3):301–12.

28. Kaibara T, Sutherland GR, Colbourne F, et al. Hypothermia: depression of tricarboxylic acid cycle flux and evidence for pentose phosphate shunt upregulation. J Neurosurg 1999;90(2):339–47.

29. Welsh FA, Sims RE, Harris VA. Mild hypothermia prevents ischemic injury in gerbil hippocampus. J Cereb Blood Flow Metab 1990;10(4):557–63.

30. Sutton LN, Clark BJ, Norwood CR, et al. Global cerebral ischemia in piglets under conditions of mild and deep hypothermia. Stroke 1991;22(12):1567–73.

31. Friedman LK, Ginsberg MD, Belayev L, et al. Intraischemic but not postischemic hypothermia prevents non-selective hippocampal downregulation of AMPA and NMDA receptor gene expression after global ischemia. Brain Res Mol Brain Res 2001;86(1–2): 34–47.

32. Mueller-Burke D, Koehler RC, Martin LJ. Rapid NMDA receptor phosphorylation and oxidative stress precede striatal neurodegeneration after hypoxic ischemia in newborn piglets and are attenuated with hypothermia. Int J Dev Neurosci 2008;26(1): 67–76.

33. Truettner JS, Alonso OF, Dietrich WD. Influence of therapeutic hypothermia on matrix metalloproteinase activity after traumatic brain injury in rats. J Cereb Blood Flow Metab 2005;25(11):1505–16.

34. Ha K-Y, Kim Y-H. Neuroprotective effect of moderate epidural hypothermia after spinal cord injury in rats. Spine 2008;33(19):2059–65.

35. Morino T, Ogata T, Takeba J, et al. Microglia inhibition is a target of mild hypothermic treatment after

the spinal cord injury. Spinal Cord 2008;46(6): 425–31.

36. Maier CM, Sun GH, Cheng D, et al. Effects of mild hypothermia on superoxide anion production, superoxide dismutase expression, and activity following transient focal cerebral ischemia. Neurobiol Dis 2002;11(1):28–42.

37. Shibuya S, Miyamoto O, Janjua NA, et al. Post-traumatic moderate systemic hypothermia reduces TUNEL positive cells following spinal cord injury in rat. Spinal Cord 2004;42(1):29–34.

38. Batchelor PE, Skeers P, Antonic A, et al. Systematic review and meta-analysis of therapeutic hypothermia in animal models of spinal cord injury. PLoS One 2013;8(8):e71317.

39. Kwon BK, Mann C, Sohn HM, et al. Hypothermia for spinal cord injury. Spine J 2008;8(6):859–74.

40. Casas CE, Herrera LP, Prusmack C, et al. Effects of epidural hypothermic saline infusion on locomotor outcome and tissue preservation after moderate thoracic spinal cord contusion in rats. J Neurosurg Spine 2005;2(3):308–18.

41. Morochovic R, Chudá M, Talánová J, et al. Local transcutaneous cooling of the spinal cord in the rat: effects on long-term outcomes after compression spinal cord injury. Int J Neurosci 2008;118(4): 555–68.

42. Dimar JR, Shields CB, Zhang YP, et al. The role of directly applied hypothermia in spinal cord injury. Spine 2000;25(18):2294–302.

43. Ok J-H, Kim Y-H, Ha K-Y. Neuroprotective effects of hypothermia after spinal cord injury in rats: comparative study between epidural hypothermia and systemic hypothermia. Spine 2012;37(25): E1551–9.

44. Maybhate A, Hu C, Bazley FA, et al. Potential long-term benefits of acute hypothermia after spinal cord injury: assessments with somatosensory-evoked potentials. Crit Care Med 2012;40(2):573–9.

45. Batchelor PE, Kerr NF, Gatt AM, et al. Hypothermia prior to decompression: buying time for treatment of acute spinal cord injury. J Neurotrauma 2010; 27(8):1357–68.

46. Duz B, Kaplan M, Bilgic S, et al. Does hypothermic treatment provide an advantage after spinal cord injury until surgery? An experimental study. Neurochem Res 2009;34(3):407–10.

47. Grulova I, Slovinska L, Nagyova M, et al. The effect of hypothermia on sensory-motor function and tissue sparing after spinal cord injury. Spine J 2013;13(12): 1881–91.

48. Lo TP, Cho K-S, Garg MS, et al. Systemic hypothermia improves histological and functional outcome after cervical spinal cord contusion in rats. J Comp Neurol 2009;514(5):433–48.

49. Karamouzian S, Akhtarshomar S, Saied A, et al. Effects of methylprednisolone on neuroprotective

effects of delay hypothermia on spinal cord injury in rat. Asian Spine J 2015;9(1):1–6.

50. Seo J-Y, Kim Y-H, Kim J-W, et al. Effects of therapeutic hypothermia on apoptosis and autophagy after spinal cord injury in rats. Spine 2015;40(12): 883–90.

51. Yu CG, Jimenez O, Marcillo AE, et al. Beneficial effects of modest systemic hypothermia on locomotor function and histopathological damage following contusion-induced spinal cord injury in rats. J Neurosurg 2000;93(1 Suppl):85–93.

52. Topuz K, Colak A, Cemil B, et al. Combined hyperbaric oxygen and hypothermia treatment on oxidative stress parameters after spinal cord injury: an experimental study. Arch Med Res 2010;41(7): 506–12.

53. Wang D, Zhang J. Effects of hypothermia combined with neural stem cell transplantation on recovery of neurological function in rats with spinal cord injury. Mol Med Rep 2015;11(3):1759–67.

54. Selker RG. Icewater irrigation of the spinal cord. Surg Forum 1971;22:411–3.

55. Tator CH. Acute spinal cord injury: a review of recent studies of treatment and pathophysiology. Can Med Assoc J 1972;107(2):143–145 passim.

56. Koons DD, Gildenberg PL, Dohn DF, et al. Local hypothermia in the treatment of spinal cord injuries. Report of seven cases. Cleve Clin Q 1972;39(3): 109–17.

57. Hansebout RR, Hansebout CR. Local cooling for traumatic spinal cord injury: outcomes in 20 patients and review of the literature. J Neurosurg Spine 2014; 20(5):550–61.

58. Tator CH, Deecke L. Value of normothermic perfusion, hypothermic perfusion, and durotomy in the treatment of experimental acute spinal cord trauma. J Neurosurg 1973;39(1):52–64.

59. Al-Senani FM, Graffagnino C, Grotta JC, et al. A prospective, multicenter pilot study to evaluate the feasibility and safety of using the CoolGard System and Icy catheter following cardiac arrest. Resuscitation 2004;62(2):143–50.

60. De Fazio C, Skrifvars MB, Søreide E, et al. Intravascular versus surface cooling for targeted temperature management after out-of-hospital cardiac arrest: an analysis of the TTH48 trial. Crit Care 2019;23(1):61.

61. Virkkunen I, Yli-Hankala A, Silfvast T. Induction of therapeutic hypothermia after cardiac arrest in prehospital patients using ice-cold Ringer's solution: a pilot study. Resuscitation 2004;62(3): 299–302.

62. Kliegel A, Losert H, Sterz F, et al. Cold simple intravenous infusions preceding special endovascular cooling for faster induction of mild hypothermia after cardiac arrest—a feasibility study. Resuscitation 2005;64(3):347–51.

63. Steinberg GK, Ogilvy CS, Shuer LM, et al. Comparison of endovascular and surface cooling during unruptured cerebral aneurysm repair. Neurosurgery 2004;55(2):307–14 [discussion 314-315].

64. Cappuccino A, Bisson LJ, Carpenter B, et al. The use of systemic hypothermia for the treatment of an acute cervical spinal cord injury in a professional football player. Spine 2010;35(2):E57–62.

65. Cappuccino A, Bisson LJ, Carpenter B, et al. Systemic hypothermia as treatment for an acute cervical spinal cord injury in a professional football player: 9-year follow-up. Am J Orthop 2017;46(2): E79–82.

66. Marino RJ, Burns S, Graves DE, et al. Upper- and lower-extremity motor recovery after traumatic cervical spinal cord injury: an update from the national spinal cord injury database. Arch Phys Med Rehabil 2011;92(3):369–75.

67. Polderman KH. Mechanisms of action, physiological effects, and complications of hypothermia. Crit Care Med 2009;37(7 Suppl):S186–202.

68. Polderman KH. Induced hypothermia and fever control for prevention and treatment of neurological injuries. Lancet 2008;371(9628):1955–69.

69. Simosa HF, Petersen DJ, Agarwal SK, et al. Increased risk of deep venous thrombosis with endovascular cooling in patients with traumatic head injury. Am Surg 2007;73(5):461–4.

70. Thompson HJ, Kirkness CJ, Mitchell PH. Hypothermia and rapid rewarming is associated with worse outcome following traumatic brain injury. J Trauma Nurs 2010;17(4):173–7.

Pharmacologic and Cell-Based Therapies for Acute Spinal Cord Injury

Nikolay L. Martirosyan, MD, PhD

KEYWORDS

- Spinal cord injury • Methylprednisolone • Riluzole • Stem cells • Cell therapy

KEY POINTS

- Methylprednisolone therapy does not provide benefit for neurologic recovery after spinal cord injury (SCI). It is associated with a higher rate of medical complications. Therefore, it should not be used in the setting of acute SCI.
- Riluzole showed potential benefit in neurologic recovery after SCI in the setting of phase I open-label trial. Results of the ongoing phase II/II trial will provide more evidence for the effect of Riluzole in patients with SCI.
- Transplantation of neural stem cells into the epicenter of SCI may result in improvement of neurologic function after SCI.

INTRODUCTION

Acute traumatic spinal cord injury (SCI) is a devastating pathology often affecting young and active individuals.[1] Despite significant scientific advances, the management of patients with SCI remains challenging. Neurologic recovery in severe cases is poor, with significant long-term morbidity affecting patients' daily life and performance. A substantial cost is associated with the lifetime management of patients with SCI.[1] Many therapeutic modalities were proposed in research laboratory settings, and few translated into clinical trials.[2-5] Here, we present a systematic review of pharmacologic and cell-based therapies to manage patients with SCI.

PHARMACOLOGIC THERAPIES
Methylprednisolone

The use of methylprednisolone (MP) for the treatment of acute SCI is the most studied therapeutic modality in humans. Several large randomized controlled multicenter trials (RCT) have been conducted to investigate the effect of MP in SCI management, including the highly regarded randomized clinical trials National Acute Spinal Cord Injury Study (NASCIS) II and III.[6-9] A number of smaller studies have also been reported.

The original NASCIS (NASCIS I) investigated low and high doses of MP following acute SCI. The high-dose group received 1000 mg of MP bolus and then daily for 10 days. The low-dose group received 100 mg of MP bolus and the daily for 10 days. A total of 306 patients were enrolled in the study. Fifty-four percent of patients were available for 6-month follow-up. No difference in neurologic recovery was identified between the 2 groups at 6 and 12 months after SCI. Patients in the high-dose MP group had a higher rate of wound complications and death.[6,10]

The NASCIS II RCT was designed to investigate the effects of MP and naloxone in the treatment of acute SCI.[9] There were 3 investigational arms: 30 mg/kg bolus of MP followed by 23-hour maintenance dose 5.4 mg/kg, 5.4 mg/kg naloxone bolus followed by 23-hour 4 mg/kg maintenance dose, and placebo group. A total of 487 patients were enrolled in this study. Naloxone did not

Department of Neurosurgery, Allen Memorial Hospital, UnityPoint Clinic, 146 W Dale Street Suite 201, Waterloo, IA 50703, USA
E-mail address: Nikolay.Martirosyan@unitypoint.org

Neurosurg Clin N Am 32 (2021) 389–395
https://doi.org/10.1016/j.nec.2021.03.010
1042-3680/21/© 2021 Elsevier Inc. All rights reserved.

show any improvement in neurologic function. The investigators reported the beneficial role of MP to improve neurologic function in patients who received treatment less than 8 hours after SCI.[11,12] However, in-depth analysis showed that these conclusions were drawn based on post hoc analyses from a much smaller cohort of patients (n = 62), likely do not represent a clinically meaningful improvement, and may in fact be due to random chance.[4] Within the entire study group of 487 patients, those who received MP had a higher rate of medical complications, including gastrointestinal bleeding, wound infection, and pulmonary embolus.[11]

Prendergast and colleagues[13] performed retrospective analysis of patients with acute SCI treated with (n = 29) and without (n = 25) MP. In this study, patients with closed SCI treated with MP did not demonstrate neurologic improvement in comparison with patients who did not receive MP. In contrast, patients with penetrating SCI treated with MP showed less improvement of neurologic status compared with controls. Gerhart and colleagues[14] performed retrospective concurrent cohort analysis. A total of 188 patients received the NASCIS II MP protocol, and 90 patients were managed without MP. There was no difference in outcomes based on Frankel grade.[14] Gerndt and colleagues[15] reported retrospective analysis of 140 patients with SCI treated with NASCIC II protocol MP. Steroid therapy was associated with a 4-fold increase in acute pneumonia and a 2.6-fold increase in the incidence of any type of pneumonia. It was also associated with increased intensive care stay and ventilator days. There was no difference in overall hospitalization length.[15]

The NASCIS III multicenter randomized double-blinded trial compared 24-hour MP (5.4 mg/h × 24 hours) administration to 48-hour MP (5.4 mg/h × 48 hours) and 48-hour tirilazad mesylate (2.5 mg/kg every 6 hours × 48 hours) in management of patients with SCI.[7,8] All patients had 30 mg/kg MP administration before randomization. There was no placebo group because the NASCIS II study reported the beneficial role of MP. A total of 499 patients were randomized in this study: 24-hour MP (n = 166), 48-hour MP (n = 166), and 48-hour tirilazad mesylate (n = 167).

Preplanned analyses of the data did not demonstrate significant differences in neurologic recovery between groups. Post hoc analysis showed statistically significant but minimal improvement in motor function in the 48-hour MP group in comparison with 24-hour MP at 6 weeks after SCI. However, this American Spinal Injury Association (ASIA) motor score difference degraded and became statistically insignificant at 1-year follow-up. Patients who received high-dose MP had a higher rate of sepsis and pneumonia.[7,8]

Pointillart and colleagues[16] conducted a prospective RCT to compare MP (NASCIS II protocol), nimodipine, and placebo to manage the acute SCI. Blinded ASIA assessment was performed at 1-year follow-up. No significant neurologic improvement was detected between groups.[16]

Matsumoto and colleagues[17] performed a prospective, randomized, and double-blind trial comparing MP (NASCIS II protocol) with placebo in patients with acute SCI within 8 hours after injury. The aim of the study was to compare complications between the groups. A total of 46 patients were enrolled, with 23 patients in each study group. Patients who received MP had a significantly higher rate of complications, including pulmonary and gastrointestinal complications.[17]

Yasuo and colleagues also performed a prospective trial to investigate the effect of MP on neurologic function after SCI. In their study, all patients with SCI for 2 consecutive years were managed with MP (NASCIS II protocol) (n = 38), and all patients following 2 consecutive years were managed without MP (n = 41). No significant difference in neurologic function was observed between groups at 3 months after SCI. Patients in the MP group had a significantly higher rate of pneumonia.[18]

Largely because of the success claimed in the NASCIS trials, for a time MP therapy became regarded as a standard of care for patients with acute SCI. However, subsequent studies and detailed reanalysis of NASCIS II and III provided evidence that MP carries a high risk of medical complications, including death, with minimal to no benefit in neurologic improvement. Although some centers continue to administer MP for the treatment of SCI, it is no longer a standard of care, and the harmful side effects are more likely to outweigh any benefit[4] (**Table 1**).

GM-1 Ganglioside

Gangliosides are a type of glycolipid and constitute a major component of cell membranes in the central nervous system. In 1991, exciting results were reported from a single institution investigating the effect of intravenous GM-1 ganglioside administration to treat SCI.[19] Sixteen patients randomized to receive the study drug showed significantly improved Frankel grades and ASIA motor scores compared with 18 patients receiving placebo. However, despite randomizing 797 patients across 28 centers, the subsequent multicenter trial failed to reproduce these results.[20] There has been

Table 1
Pharmacologic therapies for SCI in humans

Agent	Year	Design	Status	Neurologic Outcome	Comments
Methylprednisolone					
NASCIS I	1985	RCT	Published	Negative	More complications in high-dose MP group ($P < .05$)
NASCIS II	1992	RCT	Published	Negative[a]	More complications in high-dose MP group (n.s.)
NASCIS III	1998	RCT	Published	Negative[a]	More complications in the high-dose MP group (n.s.)
Prendergast	1994	retrosp cohort	Published	Negative	Neurologic deterioration when MP given in penetrating SCI ($P < .05$)
Gerhart	1995	retrosp cohort	Published	Negative	
Gerndt	1997	retrosp cohort	Published	Negative	More complications in MP group ($P < .05$)
Pointillart	2000	RCT	Published	Negative	More complications in MP group ($P < .05$)
Matsumoto	2001	RCT	Published	NT	More complications in MP group ($P < .05$)
Yasuo	2009	prosp cohort	Published	Negative	More complications in MP group ($P < .05$)
Naloxone (NASCIS II)	1992	RCT	Published	Negative	
Tirilazad (NASCIS III)	1998	RCT	Published	Negative	
Nimodipine (Pointillart)	2000	RCT	Published	Negative	
GM-1 Ganglioside	2001	RCT	Published	Negative	
Cethrin	2011	RCT	Terminated	Negative	
Minocycline	2012	RCT	Active	Pending	
Riluzole	2014	RCT	Closed	Pending	

Some post hoc analyses reported to show modest treatment effect on small subsets of the study cohort. No adjustment for multiple comparisons.

Abbreviations: MP, methylprednisolone; NASCIS, National Acute Spinal Cord Injury Study; n.s., trend observed but not statistically significant; prosp cohort, prospective cohort; RCT, randomized controlled trial; retrosp cohort, retrospective cohort; SCI, spinal cord injury.

[a] Preplanned (a priori) comparisons negative between all groups.

speculation that this subsequently negative RCT resulted from a confounding effect due to an initial steroid bolus required for all patients at the time of hospital admission (MP "standard of care"), but not included as part of the original 1991 study.

Minocycline

Minocycline is an antibiotic that has been shown to have neuroprotective effects by reducing apoptosis, microglial activation, and decreasing inflammation.[21] A phase II placebo-controlled randomized trial of minocycline was performed in acute SCI.[22] Patients were randomized into treatment (n = 27) and placebo (n = 25) groups. The treatment group patients received 7 days of intravenous minocycline. Patients in the minocycline group with cervical SCI showed a 6-point improvement in motor score in comparison with the placebo group. Patients with thoracic SCI did not show a difference in motor recovery.[22] Although these results are promising, drug availability and patient recruitment have delayed an ongoing larger multicenter trial.[23]

Rho Inhibitors

The Rho pathway is one of the important mechanisms that regulate axonal sprouting and regeneration. Laboratory studies showed that inhibition of Rho pathways with C3 transferase has a protective role for neurons from cell death after ischemia or trauma. Therefore, it is considered an appropriate target for management of SCI.[24–26] Pharmacologically synthetized C3 transferase (VX-210 AKA BA-210 aka Cethrin) was used in a clinical trial. Fehlings and colleagues[27] conducted an open-label phase I/IIa dose-escalation trial to investigate the effects of the topical extradural application of Cethrin in patients with SCI. A total of 48 patients were enrolled: 32 with a thoracic level of SCI and 16 with cervical. Five doses of medication were used: 0.3 mg, 1 mg, 3 mg, 6 mg, and 9 mg. Cethrin was applied in a mixture with fibrin sealant. ASIA assessment was performed 3, 6, and 12 months after SCI. Results demonstrated an apparent dose-response effect with higher degrees of motor improvement seen in the 3-mg group (n = 3); however, the study suffered from small numbers and lacked a control group.[27] A subsequent multi-center placebo-controlled RCT (SPRING Trial) failed its interim analysis and was terminated before completion.[28]

Riluzole

Riluzole is a benzothiazole anticonvulsant Na$^+$ channel blocker. It has been widely used in the management of patients with amyotrophic lateral sclerosis. Because of the mechanism of action, it is thought to provide a neuroprotective effect and decrease the magnitude of the secondary mechanism of SCI.[29] A phase I open-label trial investigating the safety of riluzole with secondary goals of comparing neurologic, functional, and pain outcomes has been reported in patients with SCI.[30] Fifty milligrams of riluzole was administered orally or enterally every 12 hours for 2 weeks, typically for the first 2 weeks after injury. A total of 36 patients were enrolled. An additional 36 matched patients who did not receive riluzole were selected from patient registry. Analysis of motor score recovery demonstrated improvement at 42, 90, and 180 days. ASIA Impairment Scale (AIS) grade A patients progressed from average motor scores of 16 to 31 at 180 days, grade B progressed from 16 to 60, and grade C from 32 to 82. As a phase I nonblinded safety trial, the neurologic improvement is encouraging but does not represent strong scientific evidence.[31] A phase II/III randomized, double-blinded, placebo-controlled parallel multicenter trial initiated in 2014 to further investigate role of riluzole in management of acute SCI remains active but is no longer recruiting[32] (see **Table 1**).

BIODEGRADABLE POLYMERS AS SCAFFOLDS

The concept of using a biodegradable scaffold in SCI has been widely investigated in animal models.[33,34] Scaffolds decrease scar formation and may promote axonal growth and regeneration. Recently, Kim and colleagues[35] published a clinical study evaluating implantation of bioresorbable polymer scaffold in humans with complete thoracic SCI. Nineteen patients underwent scaffold implantation. Thirteen of 16 patients experienced a change in AIS grade at 6 months; 5 patients showed improvement of the neurologic level of injury, 8 had worsening of the neurologic level of injury, and 3 patients did not improve. There were 3 serious adverse events (death) in the study, all unrelated to scaffold implantation, resulting in early termination of the study.[35] Nonetheless, varying degrees of success in animal models suggests there may eventually be a role for biodegradable scaffolds in SCI.

CELL THERAPIES

Cell transplantation is an emerging modality for the management of SCI. Numerous studies have been performed in the laboratory setting with promising results.[3,36] Safety concerns and ethical considerations are factors limiting clinical translation of these research protocols. Several small clinical trials have been reported outside of the United States and Canada using allograft transplants.[37–42] However, serious complications were linked to cell transplantation, including neoplastic conversion, infection, loss of vision, and others.[43]

Anderson and colleagues[44] reported a phase I clinical trial transplanting autologous human Schwann cells into the injury zone in patients with subacute thoracic SCI. Study patients had sural nerves harvested for Schwann cell purification and expansion. The Schwann cells were injected stereotactically into the epicenter of the thoracic SCI site. Six patients were enrolled in this study. Although no adverse events were recorded within 12 months after implantation, there were no improvements in motor function either.[44]

Levi and colleagues[45] have conducted a phase I clinical trial of intramedullary transplantation of human neural stem cells to assess safety. A total of 29 patients were enrolled. Patients did not have adverse events related to transplantation but no neurologic outcomes were reported.[45] Curtis and colleagues[46] reported neurologic improvement in patients with neural stem cell transplantation. A total of 4 patients received intramedullary transplantation of human-derived NSI-556 neural stem cells.[46] Two patients showed segmental improvement of 1 to 2 levels in both motor and sensory domains. No long-tract benefits were reported.

Cell transplantation remains in its early infancy as a therapy for SCI. Further translational research is certainly forthcoming and promises to be exciting. For a more in-depth look at the challenges and successes behind spinal cord regeneration, the reader will enjoy the article by Dr Mark Anderson on targeting central nervous system regeneration with cell type specificity, elsewhere in this issue.

SUMMARY

In summary, despite intensive basic science, animal, and human research, there currently exists no pharmacologic agent or cellular implant proven to be of benefit in treating SCI. Methylprednisolone consistently demonstrates toxicity in patients with SCI rather than benefit. Work continues, and combination therapies may hold promise. In the meantime, immobilization, blood pressure support, oxygenation, and timely decompression for incomplete injuries remain the mainstay of treatment.

CLINICS CARE POINTS

- Metyhprednisolone does not improve neurologic recovery after SCI
- Riluzole showed effectiveness in SCI
- Neural stem cells may result in neurological improvement after SCI

DISCLOSURE

The author has nothing to disclose.

REFERENCES

1. National Spinal Cord Injury Statistical Center. Spinal Cord Injury (SCI) 2016 Facts and Figures at a Glance. J Spinal Cord Med 2016;39(4):493–4.
2. Alizadeh A, Matthew DS, Karimi-Abdolrezaee S. Traumatic spinal cord injury: an overview of pathophysiology, models and acute injury mechanisms. Front Neurol 2019;10:282.
3. Assinck P, Duncan Greg J, Hilton Brett J, et al. Cell transplantation therapy for spinal cord injury. Nat Neurosci 2017. https://doi.org/10.1038/nn.4541.
4. Hurlbert RJ, Hadley MN, Walters Beverly C, et al. Pharmacological therapy for acute spinal cord injury. Neurosurgery 2015. https://doi.org/10.1227/01.neu.0000462080.04196.f7.
5. Hu XC, Lu YB, Yang YN, et al. Progress in clinical trials of cell transplantation for the treatment of spinal cord injury: How many questions remain unanswered? Neural Regen Res 2021. https://doi.org/10.4103/1673-5374.293130.
6. Bracken Michael B, Collins William F, Freeman Daniel F, et al. Efficacy of methylprednisolone in acute spinal cord injury. JAMA J Am Med Assoc 1984;251(1):45–52.
7. Bracken Michael B, Jo SM, Holford Theodore R, et al. Methylprednisolone or tirilazad mesylate administration after acute spinal cord injury: 1-year follow up: results of the third national acute spinal cord injury randomized controlled trial. J Neurosurg 1998;89(5):699–706.
8. Bracken Michael B, Shepard Mary JO, Holford Theodore R, et al. Administration of methylprednisolone for 24 or 48 hours or tirilazad mesylate for 48 hours in the treatment of acute spinal cord injury. Surv Anesthesiol 1998;42(4):1597–604.
9. Bracken Michael B, Jo SM, Collins William F, et al. A randomized, controlled trial of methylprednisolone or naloxone in the treatment of acute spinal-cord injury. N Engl J Med 1990;322(20):1405–11.
10. Bracken MB, Shepard MJ, Hellenbrand KG, et al. Methylprednisolone and neurological function 1 year after spinal cord injury. Results of the National Acute Spinal Cord Injury study. J Neurosurg 1985;63(5):704–13.
11. Bracken MB, Shepard MJ, Collins WF, et al. Methylprednisolone or naloxone treatment after acute spinal cord injury: 1-year follow-up data: results of the second National Acute Spinal Cord Injury Study. J Neurosurg 1992;76(1):23–31.
12. Bracken MB, Holford TR. Effects of timing of methylprednisolone or naloxone administration on recovery of segmental and long-tract neurological function in NASCIS 2. J Neurosurg 1993;79(4):500–7.
13. Prendergast Michael R, Saxe Jonathan M, Ledgerwood Anna M, et al. Massive steroids do not reduce the zone of injury after penetrating spinal cord injury. J Trauma 1994;37(4):576–9.
14. Gerhart Ka A, Johnson Rl L, Menconi J, et al. Utilization and effectiveness of méthylprednisolone in a population-based sample of spinal cord injured persons. Paraplegia 1995;33(6):316–21.
15. Gerndt SJ, Rodriguez JL, Pawlik JW, et al. Consequences of high-dose steroid therapy for acute spinal cord injury. J Trauma 1997;42(2):279–84.
16. Pointillart V, Petitjean Me, Wiart L, et al. Pharmacological therapy of spinal cord injury during the acute phase. Spinal Cord 2000;38(2):71–6.
17. Matsumoto T, Tamaki T, Kawakami M, et al. Early complications of high-dose methylprednisolone sodium succinate treatment in the follow-up of acute cervical spinal cord injury. Spine (Phila Pa 1976) 2001;26(4):426–30.

18. Ito Y, Sugimoto Y, Tomioka M, et al. Does high dose methylprednisolone sodium succinate really improve neurological status in patient with acute cervical cord injury?: a prospective study about neurological recovery and early complications. Spine (Phila Pa 1976) 2009;34(20):2121–4.

19. Geisler Fred H, Dorsey Frank C, Coleman William P. Recovery of motor function after spinal-cord injury — a randomized, placebo-controlled trial with GM-1 Ganglioside. N Engl J Med 1991;324(26):1829–38.

20. Geisler Fred H, Coleman William P, Giacinto G, et al. The Sygen® multicenter acute spinal cord injury study. Spine (Phila Pa 1976) 2001;26(24 SUPPL):S87–98.

21. Festoff Barry W, Syed A, Arnold Paul M, et al. Minocycline neuroprotects, reduces microgliosis, and inhibits caspase protease expression early after spinal cord injury. J Neurochem 2006;97(5):1314–26.

22. Casha S, Zygun D, McGowan MD, et al. Results of a phase II placebo-controlled randomized trial of minocycline in acute spinal cord injury. Brain 2012;135(4):1224–36.

23. Minocycline in Acute Spinal Cord Injury (MASC) - ClinicalTrials.gov. Available at: https://clinicaltrials.gov/ct2/show/NCT01828203?term=minocycline&cond=Spinal+Cord+Injuries&draw=2&rank=1. Accessed March 14, 2021.

24. Bertrand J, Winton Matthew J, Rodriguez-Hernandez N, et al. Application of Rho antagonist to neuronal cell bodies promotes neurite growth in compartmented cultures and regeneration of retinal ganglion cell axons in the optic nerve of adult rats. J Neurosci 2005;25(5):1113–21.

25. Dubreuil Catherine I, Winton Matthew J, Lisa M. Rho activation patterns after spinal cord injury and the role of activated Rho in apoptosis in the central nervous system. J Cell Biol 2003;162(2):233–43.

26. Dergham P, Benjamin E, Charles E, et al. Rho signaling pathway targeted to promote spinal cord repair. J Neurosci 2002;22(15):6570–7.

27. Fehlings Michael G, Nicholas T, James H, et al. A phase I/IIa clinical trial of a recombinant Rho protein antagonist in acute spinal cord injury. J Neurotrauma 2011;28(5):787–96.

28. Fehlings Michael G, Kim Kee D, Bizhan A, et al. Rho Inhibitor VX-210 in acute traumatic subaxial cervical spinal cord injury: design of the SPinal Cord Injury Rho INhibition InvestiGation (SPRING) Clinical Trial. J Neurotrauma 2018;35(9):1049–56.

29. Schwartz Gwen, Fehlings Michael G. Secondary injury mechanisms of spinal cord trauma: A novel therapeutic approach for the management of secondary pathophysiology with the sodium channel blocker riluzole. Prog Brain Res 2002;137.

30. Fehlings Michael G, Wilson Jefferson R, Frankowski Ralph F, et al. Riluzole for the treatment of acute traumatic spinal cord injury: rationale for and design of the NACTN Phase I clinical trial. J Neurosurg Spine 2012;17(1 Suppl):177–90.

31. Grossman Robert G, Fehlings Michael G, Frankowski Ralph F, et al. A prospective, multicenter, Phase i matched-comparison group trial of safety, pharmacokinetics, and preliminary efficacy of riluzole in patients with traumatic spinal cord injury. J Neurotrauma 2014;31(3):1049–56.

32. Riluzole in Spinal Cord Injury Study - ClinicalTrials.gov. Available at: https://clinicaltrials.gov/ct2/show/NCT01597518?term=riluzole&cond=Spinal+Cord+Injuries&draw=2&rank=1. Accessed March 14, 2021.

33. Horn Eric M, Beaumont M, Xiao ZS, et al. Influence of cross-linked hyaluronic acid hydrogels on neurite outgrowth and recovery from spinal cord injury. J Neurosurg Spine 2007;6(2):133–40.

34. Kushchayev Sergiy V, Giers Morgan B, Eng DH, et al. Hyaluronic acid scaffold has a neuroprotective effect in hemisection spinal cord injury. J Neurosurg Spine 2016;25(1):114–24.

35. Kim Kee D, Lee KS, Coric D, et al. A study of probable benefit of a bioresorbable polymer scaffold for safety and neurological recovery in patients with complete thoracic spinal cord injury: 6-month results from the INSPIRE study. J Neurosurg Spine 2021. https://doi.org/10.3171/2020.8.spine191507.

36. Hojjat-Allah A, Somayeh N, Shahram D, et al. Stem cell transplantation and functional recovery after spinal cord injury: a systematic review and meta-analysis. Anat Cell Biol 2018;51(3):180–8.

37. Dai G, Liu X, Zhang Z, et al. Transplantation of autologous bone marrow mesenchymal stem cells in the treatment of complete and chronic cervical spinal cord injury. Brain Res 2013;1533:73–9.

38. Chan RJ, Seob SI, Han KS, et al. Safety of intravenous infusion of human adipose tissue-derived mesenchymal stem cells in animals and humans. Stem Cells Dev 2011;20(8):1297–308.

39. Mackay-Sim A, Féron F, Cochrane J, et al. Autologous olfactory ensheathing cell transplantation in human paraplegia: A 3-year clinical trial. Brain 2008;131(9):2376–86.

40. Chernykh ER, Stupak VV, Muradov GM, et al. Application of autologous bone marrow stem cells in the therapy of spinal cord injury patients. Bull Exp Biol Med 2007;143(4):543–7.

41. Yoon SH, Shim YS, Park YH, et al. Complete spinal cord injury treatment using autologous bone marrow cell transplantation and bone marrow stimulation with granulocyte macrophage-colony stimulating factor: phase I/II Clinical Trial. Stem Cells 2007;25(8):2066–73.

42. Mendonca MVP, Larocca TF, de Freitas Souza BS, et al. Safety and neurological assessments after autologous transplantation of bone marrow mesenchymal stem cells in subjects with chronic spinal cord injury. Stem Cell Res Ther 2014;5(6):126.

43. Bauer G, Elsallab M, Abou-El-Enein M. Concise review: a comprehensive analysis of reported adverse events in patients receiving unproven stem cell-based interventions. Stem Cells Transl Med 2018; 7:676–85.
44. Anderson Kim D, Guest James D, Dalton DW, et al. Safety of autologous human schwann cell transplantation in subacute thoracic spinal cord injury. J Neurotrauma 2017;34(21):2950–63.
45. Levi Allan D, Okonkwo David O, Park P, et al. Emerging safety of intramedullary transplantation of human neural stem cells in chronic cervical and thoracic spinal cord injury. Clin Neurosurg 2018; 82(4):562–75.
46. Curtis E, Martin Joel R, Gabel B, et al. A first-in-human, phase i study of neural stem cell transplantation for chronic spinal cord injury. Cell Stem Cell 2018;22(6):941–50.e6.

Targeting Central Nervous System Regeneration with Cell Type Specificity

Mark A. Anderson, PhD[a,b],*

KEYWORDS

- Spinal cord injury • Neuronal regeneration • Neural repair • Growth programs

KEY POINTS

- Axon regeneration is required for functional recovery following severe spinal cord injury.
- Functional recovery mediated by axon regeneration is not robust.
- Central nervous system (CNS) neurons are heterogeneous and possess multiple subtypes.
- A greater understanding of subtype-specific regenerative responses is needed.

INTRODUCTION

Spinal cord injury (SCI) lesions are broadly classified as either incomplete or complete. Incomplete SCI lesions spare surrounding neural tissue and residual axon projections. This spared tissue is capable of rescuing varying degrees of lost function, which is augmented through rehabilitation training in animals[1–3] and humans.[4–8] Conversely, complete injuries spare little to no neural tissue, resulting in permanent and irreversible loss of motor, autonomic, and sensory functions for which rehabilitation is not effective. It is universally agreed that biologic repair is necessary to reconstruct damaged circuits and restore lost function.

Understanding why central nervous system (CNS) axons fail to regrow following injury and developing repair strategies to overcome this failure has been a heavily studied topic for much of the past century. Pioneering work in the 1980s by Aguayo and colleagues[9–11] reported that CNS axons could be coaxed to regrow into peripheral nerve grafts. This suggested two things: the environment of the mature CNS is not supportive to axon regrowth, and the CNS environment created by trauma is devoid of growth supportive factors that are required for axon regrowth.

Research in the 1980s to 2000s focused heavily on identifying and trying to neutralize potential inhibitory molecules around CNS lesions and associated with degenerating myelin.[12–15] This was followed by work on digesting chondroitin sulfate proteoglycans, which were reported to be potent inhibitors of axon growth in vitro and are present around lesion sites and engulf perineuronal nets in the gray matter.[16,17] Although neutralizing inhibition was initially hoped to be a singular solution to axon regeneration, it has not held the test of time and replication, although its effect on axon sprouting has been well documented.[16,18,19] The search for other factors involved in suppressing regeneration led to the identification and manipulation of several growth-repressing signaling pathways[20–22] and growth factors[23–25] whose augmentation resulted in impressive degrees of axon regeneration. As discussed in more detail later, these technologies have transformed the field. It is now clear that promoting successful axon regeneration through regions of injury involves modulation of the traumatic environment and increasing neuronal regenerative capacity. Yet, despite impressive axon regeneration in models of severe SCI, robust functional recovery is lacking. Exactly what is missing remains to be

[a] Brain Mind Institute, Faculty of Life Sciences, École Polytechnique Féderale de Lausanne (EPFL), Lausanne, Switzerland; [b] Neural Repair Unit, NeuroRestore, Department of Clinical Neuroscience, Lausanne University Hospital (CHUV) and University of Lausanne (UNIL), Lausanne, Switzerland
* Campus Biotech, Chemin des Mines 9, 1202 Geneva, Switzerland.
E-mail address: mark.anderson@epfl.ch

Neurosurg Clin N Am 32 (2021) 397–405
https://doi.org/10.1016/j.nec.2021.03.011

discovered. This review outlines the neuropathologic response to SCI and argues that a more nuanced understanding of neuron subtype-specific regenerative responses is needed to mediate biologic repair capable of restoring lost functions.

PATHOLOGY: CELLULAR AND MOLECULAR RESPONSES TO SPINAL CORD INJURY

The pathologic response to SCI consists of the immediate mechanical injury of the spinal cord, followed by a secondary phase that takes place shortly thereafter, evolves over a period of months, and comprises a series of biochemical and cellular events.[26] The initial injury, generally in the form of compression or laceration of the spinal cord, is followed by an immediate immune response, subsequent cell proliferation, scar formation, and tissue remodeling.[27] During the immediate inflammatory phase, cells within the lesion die from internally programmed suicide (apoptosis), and neurons go through Wallerian degeneration, whereby axons "die-back" from the lesion (**Fig. 1**A). Axons at the epicenter of the injury are transected, whereas those in the periphery become demyelinated. During the initial inflammatory phase, various molecules and then cells penetrate the injury site to begin the process of debris clearance. Blood-borne molecules are the first to infiltrate and signal to local cells to produce components of the extracellular matrix, such as laminins, fibronectins, and collagens, which then function as a scaffold by which inflammatory macrophages then enter.

Cell proliferation begins approximately 2 days postinjury and leads to the formation of the fibrotic scar and surrounding astroglial scar-border. Fibrotic scar is formed by the proliferation of non-neural cells including endogenous fibroblasts, pericytes, and endothelial cells that occupy the central compartment of CNS lesions,[28] whereas the astrocyte scar-border serves to demarcate areas of damaged tissue and to sequester viable (neural tissue) from nonviable (fibrotic) tissue.[29–31] The end result of this scarring segregates the spinal cord lesion into three major lesion compartments: (1) the central lesion cavity, referred to as the nonneural lesion core or fibrotic scar; (2) the surrounding astroglial scar-border; and (3) a region of spared but reactive and reorganizing neural tissue[27,32,33] (see **Fig. 1**A). The following sections discuss in more detail astrocyte scar-border and fibrotic scar formation, and highlight some of the challenges these are thought to present in regards to axon regeneration.

CELL REACTIVITY: ASTROCYTE SCAR-BORDER FORMATION

Astrocytes are a type of glial cell that tile the entire CNS, where they occupy individual, nonoverlapping territories and assist in maintaining normal circuit function. Long thought to be mere support cells for neurons, astrocytes have now been implicated in almost every facet of neurologic function.

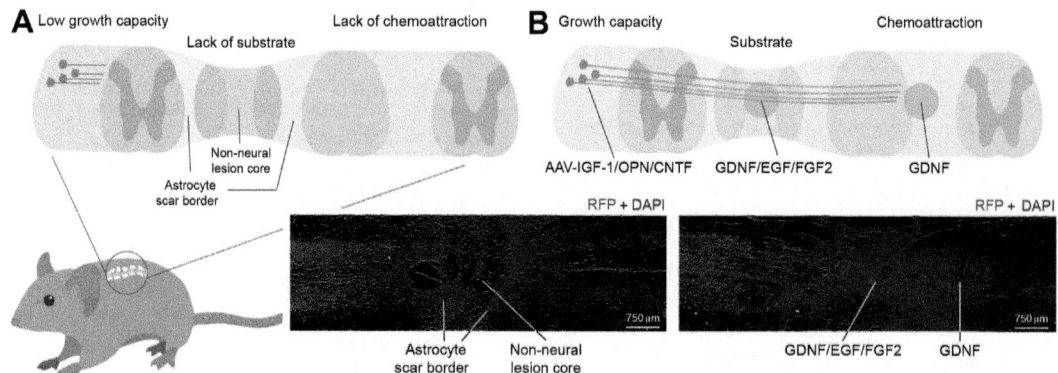

Fig. 1. Axon regeneration after SCI. (*A*) Scheme depicts axon regenerative failure following SCI. The nonneural lesion core is surrounded by an astrocyte scar border that demarcates damaged tissue from reactive and remodeling neural tissue that has been spared from the injury. Axons fail to regrow because of a combined lack of (1) neuronal growth capacity, (2) supportive substrate, and (3) chemoattraction. Photomicrograph depicts RFP-labeled propriospinal axons stopping at the lesion scar border. (*B*) Scheme depicts biologic repair strategy that targets (1) upregulation of intrinsic neuronal growth capacity by viral overexpression of IGF-1/OPN/CNTF, (2) upregulation of supportive substrate via biomaterial delivery of EGF/FGF2, and (3) chemoattraction via biomaterial delivery of GDNF. Photomicrograph depicts RFP-labeled propriospinal axons growing into and through nonneural lesion cores and toward chemoattractant below the lesion.

Astrocytes are widely known for their response to injury and disease, which they respond to with a process referred to as astrogliosis. Previously believed to be a homogeneous and detrimental event resulting in scar formation, evidence gathered over the past 30 years has demonstrated the contrary.[34] It is now clear that astrogliosis is not a single uniform event, but is a highly heterogeneous process that depends largely on the severity and type of CNS insult. At the lower end of the spectrum, mild to moderate astrogliosis results in cell hypertrophy and changes in gene expression that are reversible and subside over time. Severe astrogliosis, such as what occurs after SCI, results in cell proliferation, scar-border formation, and permanent tissue reorganization. This is a major and well-studied pathology of many neurodegenerative diseases and is a prominent feature of SCI.[16,31,32,35]

Transgenic and genomic techniques have allowed progress to be made in understanding the mechanisms of astrocyte function and scar-border formation. Following severe CNS insults, astrocytes divide and form a dense meshwork of interwoven cells surrounding the lesion perimeter. Scar-border-forming astrocytes do not migrate from other areas of the CNS, but rather derive from newly proliferated astrocytes located at and near the injury site. There has been some controversy suggesting that scar-border-forming astrocytes originate from ependymal cells located in the central canal.[36,37] However, recent work has reported that when the ependyma is not directly severed, ependymal cells contribute extremely minimally to astrocyte scar-border formation.[38]

Loss of function studies have demonstrated that the role of astrocyte scar-border formation is to seal off the lesion area to prevent inflammation from further damaging areas of healthy tissue. Preventing or attenuating astrocyte scar-border formation results in increased inflammation, cell death, demyelination, and worsened behavioral recovery.[29,30,35] However, this protective function has long been balanced by the widespread belief that scar-border formation is a key contributor to regenerative failure. The notion of astrocyte-mediated inhibition was initially caused by its barrier-like appearance and was further propagated by reports that astrocytes upregulate chondroitin sulfate proteoglycans, which inhibit axon growth in vitro and in vivo.[16,39]

Recent evidence supports the notion that scar-border-forming astrocytes may not be the primary inhibitor to axon regrowth that they were once thought. Loss-of-function studies have directly tested this hypothesis and have reported that attenuation or ablation of scar-border-forming astrocytes does not result in spontaneous axon regeneration. Rather, when intrinsic neuronal growth capacity is stimulated and chemoattractive growth factors are provided, the formation of the astroglial scar-border in fact supports the regrowth of regenerating sensory axons into non-neuronal SCI lesion cores.[31] Preventing or attenuating astrocyte scar-border formation also attenuates this stimulated regeneration. This similar concept has also been found to be true for propriospinal axons (**Fig. 1**B),[25] suggesting that the growth-supportive nature of scar-border-forming astrocytes is likely beneficial for most if not all types of CNS axons.

CELL REACTIVITY: FIBROTIC SCAR FORMATION

Considerably less attention has been given to the fibrotic component of the scar. However, recent studies have highlighted the inhibitory nature of the fibrotic scar,[20,40,41] which document regenerating axons specifically avoiding areas of fibrotic tissue. Mechanistic information regarding the origin and function of the fibrotic scar is gradually accumulating.

Following CNS injury, fibroblasts from locally damaged meninges are recruited by macrophages and then migrate into the lesion site where they proliferate and form the fibrotic scar.[42] The fibrotic scar is characterized by an array of nonneural cells (predominantly fibroblast-lineage cells, endothelia, fibrocytes, pericytes, and inflammatory cells) and these produce extracellular matrix molecules. Similar to the astrocytic scar-border, this fibrotic component is thought to serve protective and detrimental roles following CNS injury. It protects nearby tissue and assists in resealing the blood brain barrier (BBB).[43] However, it is also believed to be inhibitory for axon growth.[27,44] Fibroblasts have been reported to express multiple inhibitors of axon growth, including NG2, phosphacan, tenascin-C, semaphorin 3A, and EphB2. Strategies targeting the attenuation of fibrotic scar have reported beneficial results.

The microtubule stabilizing pharmacologic compounds taxol[45] and epothilone B[46] have been reported to reduce fibrotic scar formation, which was correlated with enhanced sensory and serotonergic axon innervation and functional recovery following SCI.[45] Another interesting study[47] reported that moderate reduction of type A pericyte scar formation results in less extracellular matrix deposition and enhanced regrowth of corticospinal tract (CST) and RST: reticulospinal tract (RST) axons into and around SCI lesions, resulting in increased electrophysiologic connectivity and functional recovery. This suggests that it may be possible to achieve functional axon regeneration in the absence of promoting neuronal growth capacity. However, therapeutic strategies targeting fibrotic scar need to strike a delicate balance between mild to moderate attenuation, because too much attenuation has been reported to cause the failure of wound healing and expand the injury site, negatively impacting neural repair and functional recovery.[37,47,48]

NEURONAL HETEROGENEITY: LESSONS FROM THE OPTIC NERVE

CNS neurons are distinct in their morphology, physiology, gene expression, and function. Furthermore, different neuronal subtypes display heterogeneous regenerative responses and possess specific activation requirements.[25,49,50] A comprehensive understanding of the molecular architecture of CNS neurons is pivotal to devising targeted regenerative strategies to manipulate their growth. Retinal ganglion cells (RGCs) have been extensively characterized, and their mechanistic dissection over the past several decades provides an ideal conceptual framework that would be beneficial to apply to other CNS neurons.

Survival or Death

Before a neuron can regenerate, it must first survive axotomy. Work initially performed by David Aguayo's group[51] demonstrated that most (>80%) RGCs die following axotomy, and that this is at least partially caused by a lack of neurotropic support. RGC survival is enhanced via exogeneous delivery of brain-derived neurotrophic factor,[52] and axon sprouting is enhanced with certain growth factors.[53] This principle has been

subsequently confirmed for corticospinal neurons[54,55] and spinal motor neurons,[56,57] where specific growth factors, but not others, enhance their survival following axotomy. Survival correlates with the distance of the neuronal soma from the site of axotomy. This may partially explain why most RGCs die following optic nerve crush,[52] and some short propriospinal neurons following SCI,[58] whereas long descending propriospinal,[58] corticospinal, and rubrospinal neurons[59,60] have been reported to survive following axotomy at the spinal level. Although some neurons respond to particular growth factors, this is dependent on the level of receptor expression in the soma, and neurons vary in the degree to which they express specific receptors.[54] A more thorough understanding of growth factor receptor expression levels across cell types is needed to develop targeted repair strategies (**Fig. 2**).

The recent revolution in single cell RNA sequencing has revealed multiple and previously unknown types of neurons within the optic nerve[61,62] and spinal cord.[63–65] More than 40 transcriptionally distinct types of RGC have been identified, and their ability to survive or die following axotomy varies greatly among subtypes. Although most RGCs that survive are αRGCs, certain subtypes of these also die, suggesting that factors beyond transcriptional proximity contribute to survival ability.[61] Although there are some correlative similarities in cellular morphology and physiology among surviving RGCs, no single factor predicted survival, suggesting that even within subtypes that survived, they did so via differing mechanisms. Recent advances in the analysis of bioinformatic datasets may prove valuable in prioritizing cell types based on their ability to respond to experimental perturbations,[66] and their development

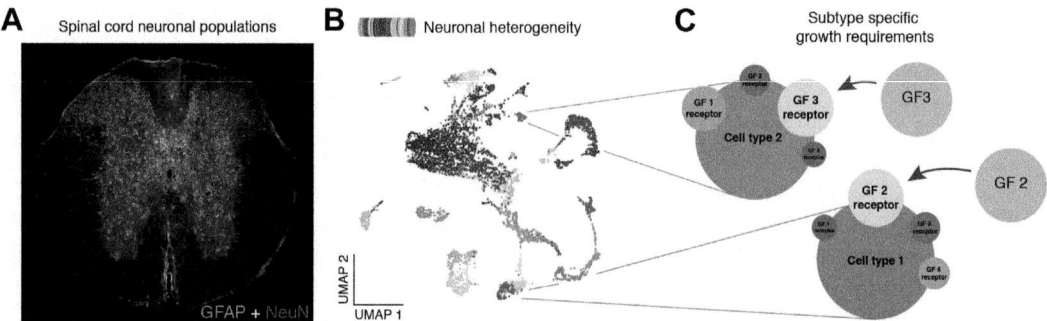

Fig. 2. Neuronal heterogeneity and subtype-specific activation requirements. (*A*) Photomicrograph depicting spinal cord neuronal populations on a cross-section of mouse spinal cord tissue immunohistochemically stained for GFAP (*green*) and NeuN (*red*). (*B*) Uniform manifold approximation and projection (UMAP) visualization of single-nucleus sequencing of mouse spinal cord neurons depicting more than 40 transcriptionally distinct neuronal subtypes. (*C*) Scheme depicting how different neurons within the spinal cord may have different receptors for specific growth factors (GF) to induce their regeneration.

and widespread use will shed light on how heterogeneous cellular populations respond to experimental manipulations and will be instrumental in guiding cell specific repair strategies.

Influencing Regeneration

Although several neurotropic factors (brain-derived neurotrophic factor, glial derived neurotrophic factor (GDNF), Ciliary neurotrophic factor (CNTF), and fibroblast growth factor-1 [FGF-1]) aid in promoting neuronal survival, most have classically failed at promoting any meaningful regeneration.[67] Nonetheless, some axons regenerate into peripheral nerve grafts,[11,68] suggesting a limited degree of growth capacity is maintained. RGCs undergo a developmental decline in their regenerative ability and adult RGCs do not extend axons by default but require the presence of neurotropic cues.[67,69–71] Various factors have been identified that promote a degree of regeneration, including zymosan,[67] angiotensin II,[72] and others, and combining these with peripheral nerve grafts further potentiates this growth.

Although initial successes in RGC regeneration seemed promising, the overall growth was modest.[72] Similar findings proved true in the context of SCI, where a combination of permissive cell grafts and neurotropic factors elicited a limited degree of regenerative growth.[9,49,73,74] Nonetheless, in both injury models and in all types of neurons studied, it was abundantly clear that an increase in growth by several orders of magnitude would be required to achieve a clinically meaningful result capable of restoring lost function.

Elegant work from Zhigang He's laboratory spearheaded the discovery and application of factors regulating intrinsic neuronal growth programs. Numerous molecular regulators of axon growth have been and continue to be identified. An in-depth discussion of these is beyond the scope of this review and has been discussed elsewhere.[75–77] Briefly, deletion of PTEN,[78] SOCS3,[79] c-myc,[80] DCLK,[81] and members of the KLF family[82] have been reported to robustly increase the amount of regeneration of RGCs following optic nerve crush, and combinations of these manipulations have been reported to further augment this growth.[21,80] Recent work has led to the identification of different combinations of growth factors, such as Insulin-like growth factor-1 (IGF-1), osteopontin (OPN), and CNTF, which act on similar molecular pathways and yield similar degrees of regeneration,[23–25,50] a key step toward eventual clinical translation.

Nevertheless, although these manipulations result in extensive regeneration, they do not act on all types of neurons equally, and subtype-specific responses have emerged.[25,50,83] PTEN deletion results in the survival and regeneration of RGCs following axotomy, but is restricted primarily to αRGCs, which constitute just 6% of the total RGC population.[50] PTEN acts by elevating mTOR activity, which declines following development. αRGCs have naturally high levels of mTOR activity, and this may partially explain their robust growth response in comparison with other types of RGCs. Forced overexpression of the growth factors OPN and IGF-1 results in a similar degree of regeneration as PTEN deletion, and αRGCs selectively express receptors for both these growth factors. Together, these findings suggest that signaling pathways regulating growth are not uniform among CNS neurons, or even among subtypes of the same class of neuron. Finding the appropriate permutations to elicit a more comprehensive regenerative response across RGC subtypes requires a highly nuanced understanding of the specific signaling pathways regulating subtype-specific growth, and needs to be balanced by positive and negative effects different perturbations may have. For example, overexpression of the transcription factor Sox11 results in the death of αRGCs, but in the regeneration of non-αRGCs.[83] Although more work needs to be done in this area, it is intriguing to imagine that given the limited amount of neurons currently capable of regenerating, the field has only seen a fraction of what is theoretically possible.

NEURONAL HETEROGENEITY: APPLICATION TO SPINAL CORD INJURY

Most effective manipulations currently applied to SCI were initially discovered from studies in the optic nerve. Compared with the eye, these manipulations are not as effective in the context of SCI, likely caused by differing lesion pathologies. Although lesions to the optic nerve result in a spared contiguous bridge of reactive astroglia along which regenerating axons grow across, severe and complete SCI lesions often do not have spared tissue bridges, and the nonsupportive nature of the fibrotic scar poses a significant barrier to regeneration.

SCI lesions are grafted with various cells, and combining these with delivery of neurotropic factors results in some growth of ascending and descending axons into grafts.[49] Similar to findings from the optic nerve, all neurons do not regenerate equally, and observations of heterogeneous growth responses are emerging. A traditional belief is that corticospinal neurons are the most refractory to regeneration, whereas dorsal root ganglion neurons and raphespinal (serotonergic) neurons the most responsive to regeneration. This idea, however, is largely based on spontaneous and correlative growth responses, where corticospinal axons die back considerably, whereas serotonergic and sensory axons remain in close proximity to lesion borders.[31]

The notion of refractory versus responsive regeneration may be somewhat misguided. Emerging evidence suggests the issue lies more in dissecting appropriate requirements to trigger the regenerative programs of different subtypes of neuron. Although corticospinal neurons are considered the most refractory type of CNS neuron, PTEN deletion results in robust regrowth of corticospinal[20,22] axons following SCI, but is ineffective at promoting propriospinal axon growth,[25] which are considered to have a naturally high regenerative capacity.[84] Currently, a manipulation that induces robust regrowth from multiple tracts, including the corticospinal tract, is grafts of caudalized neural stem cells.[85,86] This is achieved partially by transforming the regenerating corticospinal neuron to an embryonic transcriptional state,[87] but the exact mechanisms of how the neuron regenerates, or what neurotropic cues are secreted by the graft, are not known.

Chemoattraction and growth factor specificity have also become recognized as important elements in overcoming regenerative failure. Achieving regeneration of propriospinal[25] and sensory[31] axons into nonneural lesion cores requires the presence of chemoattractive cues in combination with upregulation of intrinsic neuronal growth programs. Propriospinal neurons, activated by overexpression of IGF-1, OPN, and CNTF and chemoattracted by GDNF, grow robustly into and through SCI lesions (see **Fig. 1**B), whereas 5HT neurons do not.[25] This suggests that a major issue to solving regeneration lies in finding the right combination of factors that are specific to the cell population being studied (see **Fig. 2**C).

Although the field of SCI has made tremendous advances in achieving regeneration, the normalized percentage of regeneration relative to an intact spinal cord is still modest. The reason for this is not clear. One likely reason is that, similar to RGC neurons in the optic nerve, supraspinal and intraspinal neurons comprise a heterogeneous mix of cells that likely respond differently to growth factors and transcriptional manipulations. It has been reported that there are more than 40 different types of neurons in the lumbar spinal cord of the adult mouse,[64] and each of these subtypes vary in growth factor receptor levels (see **Fig. 2**A–C). Exploiting single cell technology to identify genetic programs that drive

regeneration is important in finding candidate molecules or growth factors that can be used to target different neuron subtypes.

SUMMARY

There is now compelling evidence suggesting that different neuronal subtypes display heterogeneous regenerative responses and possess specific activation requirements. Although the level of regeneration currently achievable is impressive, it fails to yield robust functional recovery. Given what is known about cellular heterogeneity, current strategies are likely biased to cell types with a particular transcriptomic profile. More information on growth programs within specific neuronal populations is required to overcome this barrier to growth. Going forward, it will be useful to develop a deeper and more nuanced understanding of the genetic and functional diversity that exists within the numerous populations of CNS neurons. This will enable researchers to create tailored and cell type–specific regenerative interventions that have the potential to restore functions lost through SCI.

CLINICS CARE POINTS

- Biological repair strategies which stimulate axon regrowth across lesion sites will be key to allowing recovery of function following severe SCI.
- Currently, no such strategies exist for human patients with SCI.
- The requirements to achieve regeneration among different types of neurons are not the same, and a in depth dissection of these regeneration requirements will be necessary to foster functional recovery following severe SCI.

ACKNOWLEDGMENTS

The author thanks Matthieu Gautier for design of the figures, and Jordan Squair for useful discussions.

DISCLOSURE

M.A.A is supported by a SNF Ambizione fellowship (PZ00P3_185728) and the ALARME Foundation (531066).

REFERENCES

1. Asboth L, Friedli L, Beauparlant J, et al. Cortico-reticulo-spinal circuit reorganization enables functional recovery after severe spinal cord contusion. Nat Neurosci 2018;21(4):576–88.
2. van den Brand R, Heutschi J, Barraud Q, et al. Restoring voluntary control of locomotion after paralyzing spinal cord injury. Science 2012;336(6085):1182–5.
3. Courtine G, Gerasimenko Y, van den Brand R, et al. Transformation of nonfunctional spinal circuits into functional states after the loss of brain input. Nat Neurosci 2009;12(10):1333–42.
4. Harkema S, Gerasimenko Y, Hodes J, et al. Effect of epidural stimulation of the lumbosacral spinal cord on voluntary movement, standing, and assisted stepping after motor complete paraplegia: a case study. Lancet 2011;377(9781):1938–47.
5. Angeli CA, Boakye M, Morton RA, et al. Recovery of over-ground walking after chronic motor complete spinal cord injury. N Engl J Med 2018;379(13):1244–50.
6. Angeli CA, Edgerton VR, Gerasimenko YP, et al. Altering spinal cord excitability enables voluntary movements after chronic complete paralysis in humans. Brain 2014;137(Pt 5):1394–409.
7. Wagner FB, Mignardot J-B, Le Goff-Mignardot CG, et al. Targeted neurotechnology restores walking in humans with spinal cord injury. Nature 2018;563(7729):65–71.
8. Gill ML, Grahn PJ, Calvert JS, et al. Neuromodulation of lumbosacral spinal networks enables independent stepping after complete paraplegia. Nat Med 2018. https://doi.org/10.1038/s41591-018-0175-7.
9. David S, Aguayo AJ. Axonal elongation into peripheral nervous system "bridges" after central nervous system injury in adult rats. Science 1981;214(4523):931–3.
10. Benfey M, Aguayo AJ. Extensive elongation of axons from rat brain into peripheral nerve grafts. Nature 1982;296(5853):150–2.
11. Richardson PM, McGuinness UM, Aguayo AJ. Axons from CNS neurons regenerate into PNS grafts. Nature 1980;284(5753):264–5.
12. Gonzenbach RR, Schwab ME. Disinhibition of neurite growth to repair the injured adult CNS: focusing on Nogo. Cell Mol Life Sci 2008;65(1):161–76.
13. Schwab ME, Caroni P. Antibody against myelin-associated inhibitor of neurite growth neutralizes nonpermissive substrate properties of CNS white matter. Neuron 2008;60(3):404–5.
14. Schnell L, Schwab ME. Axonal regeneration in the rat spinal cord produced by an antibody against myelin-associated neurite growth inhibitors. Nature 1990;343(6255):269–72.
15. Zheng B, Atwal J, Ho C, et al. Genetic deletion of the Nogo receptor does not reduce neurite inhibition in vitro or promote corticospinal tract regeneration in vivo. Proc Natl Acad Sci U S A 2005;102(4):1205–10.
16. Silver J, Miller JH. Regeneration beyond the glial scar. Nat Rev Neurosci 2004;5(2):146–56.
17. Bradbury EJ, Moon LDF, Popat RJ, et al. Chondroitinase ABC promotes functional recovery after spinal cord injury. Nature 2002;416(6881):636–40.
18. Lang BT, Cregg JM, DePaul MA, et al. Modulation of the proteoglycan receptor PTPsigma promotes recovery after spinal cord injury. Nature 2015;518(7539):404–8.
19. Bartus K, James ND, Didangelos A, et al. Large-scale chondroitin sulfate proteoglycan digestion with chondroitinase gene therapy leads to reduced pathology and modulates macrophage phenotype following spinal cord contusion injury. J Neurosci 2014;34(14):4822–36.
20. Zukor K, Belin S, Wang C, et al. Short hairpin RNA against PTEN enhances regenerative growth of corticospinal tract axons after spinal cord injury. J Neurosci 2013;33(39):15350–61.
21. Sun F, Park KK, Belin S, et al. Sustained axon regeneration induced by co-deletion of PTEN and SOCS3. Nature 2011;480(7377):372–5.
22. Liu K, Lu Y, Lee JK, et al. PTEN deletion enhances the regenerative ability of adult corticospinal neurons. Nat Neurosci 2010;13(9):1075–81.
23. Bei F, Lee HHC, Liu X, et al. Restoration of visual function by enhancing conduction in regenerated axons. Cell 2016;164(1–2):219–32.
24. Liu Y, Wang X, Li W, et al. A sensitized IGF1 treatment restores corticospinal axon-dependent functions. Neuron 2017;95(4):817–33.e4.
25. Anderson MA, O'Shea TM, Burda JE, et al. Required growth facilitators propel axon regeneration across complete spinal cord injury. Nature 2018;561(7723):396–400.
26. Squair JW, Tigchelaar S, Moon K-M, et al. Integrated systems analysis reveals conserved gene networks underlying response to spinal cord injury. Elife 2018;7. https://doi.org/10.7554/eLife.39188.
27. Burda JE, Sofroniew MV. Reactive gliosis and the multicellular response to CNS damage and disease. Neuron 2014;81(2):229–48.
28. Fernández-Klett F, Priller J. The fibrotic scar in neurological disorders. Brain Pathol 2014;24(4):404–13.
29. Faulkner JR, Herrmann JE, Woo MJ, et al. Reactive astrocytes protect tissue and preserve function after spinal cord injury. J Neurosci 2004;24(9):2143–55.
30. Herrmann JE, Imura T, Song B, et al. STAT3 is a critical regulator of astrogliosis and scar formation after spinal cord injury. J Neurosci 2008;28(28):7231–43.

31. Anderson MA, Burda JE, Ren Y, et al. Astrocyte scar formation aids central nervous system axon regeneration. Nature 2016;532(7598):195–200.

32. Sofroniew MV. Dissecting spinal cord regeneration. Nature 2018;557(7705):343–50.

33. O'Shea TM, Burda JE, Sofroniew MV. Cell biology of spinal cord injury and repair. J Clin Invest 2017; 127(9):3259–70.

34. Anderson MA, Ao Y, Sofroniew MV. Heterogeneity of reactive astrocytes. Neurosci Lett 2014;565:23–9.

35. Wanner IB, Anderson MA, Song B, et al. Glial scar borders are formed by newly proliferated, elongated astrocytes that interact to corral inflammatory and fibrotic cells via STAT3-dependent mechanisms after spinal cord injury. J Neurosci 2013;33(31): 12870–86.

36. Meletis K, Barnabé-Heider F, Carlén M, et al. Spinal cord injury reveals multilineage differentiation of ependymal cells. PLoS Biol 2008;6(7):e182.

37. Sabelström H, Stenudd M, Réu P, et al. Resident neural stem cells restrict tissue damage and neuronal loss after spinal cord injury in mice. Science 2013;342(6158):637–40.

38. Ren Y, Ao Y, O'Shea TM, et al. Ependymal cell contribution to scar formation after spinal cord injury is minimal, local and dependent on direct ependymal injury. Sci Rep 2017;7:41122.

39. Davies SJ, Fitch MT, Memberg SP, et al. Regeneration of adult axons in white matter tracts of the central nervous system. Nature 1997;390(6661): 680–3.

40. Schreiber J, Schachner M, Schumacher U, et al. Extracellular matrix alterations, accelerated leukocyte infiltration and enhanced axonal sprouting after spinal cord hemisection in tenascin-C-deficient mice. Acta Histochem 2013;115(8):865–78.

41. Soderblom C, Luo X, Blumenthal E, et al. Perivascular fibroblasts form the fibrotic scar after contusive spinal cord injury. J Neurosci 2013;33(34):13882–7.

42. Zhu Y, Soderblom C, Krishnan V, et al. Hematogenous macrophage depletion reduces the fibrotic scar and increases axonal growth after spinal cord injury. Neurobiol Dis 2015;74:114–25.

43. Kawano H, Kimura-Kuroda J, Komuta Y, et al. Role of the lesion scar in the response to damage and repair of the central nervous system. Cell Tissue Res 2012;349(1):169–80.

44. Hermanns S, Klapka N, Gasis M, et al. The collagenous wound healing scar in the injured central nervous system inhibits axonal regeneration. Adv Exp Med Biol 2006;557:177–90.

45. Hellal F, Hurtado A, Ruschel J, et al. Microtubule stabilization reduces scarring and causes axon regeneration after spinal cord injury. Science 2011; 331(6019):928–31.

46. Ruschel J, Hellal F, Flynn KC, et al. Axonal regeneration. Systemic administration of epothilone B promotes axon regeneration after spinal cord injury. Science 2015;348(6232):347–52.

47. Dias DO, Kim H, Holl D, et al. Reducing pericyte-derived scarring promotes recovery after spinal cord injury. Cell 2018;173(1):153–65.e22.

48. Göritz C, Dias DO, Tomilin N, et al. A pericyte origin of spinal cord scar tissue. Science 2011;333(6039): 238–42.

49. Assinck P, Duncan GJ, Hilton BJ, et al. Cell transplantation therapy for spinal cord injury. Nat Neurosci 2017;20(5):637–47.

50. Duan X, Qiao M, Bei F, et al. Subtype-specific regeneration of retinal ganglion cells following axotomy: effects of osteopontin and mTOR signaling. Neuron 2015;85(6):1244–56.

51. Villegas-Pérez MP, Vidal-Sanz M, Bray GM, et al. Influences of peripheral nerve grafts on the survival and regrowth of axotomized retinal ganglion cells in adult rats. J Neurosci 1988;8(1):265–80.

52. Mansour-Robaey S, Clarke DB, Wang YC, et al. Effects of ocular injury and administration of brain-derived neurotrophic factor on survival and regrowth of axotomized retinal ganglion cells. Proc Natl Acad Sci U S A 1994;91(5):1632–6.

53. Sawai H, Clarke DB, Kittlerova P, et al. Brain-derived neurotrophic factor and neurotrophin-4/5 stimulate growth of axonal branches from regenerating retinal ganglion cells. J Neurosci 1996;16(12):3887–94.

54. Giehl KM, Tetzlaff W. BDNF and NT-3, but not NGF, prevent axotomy-induced death of rat corticospinal neurons in vivo. Eur J Neurosci 1996;8(6):1167–75.

55. Hollis ER 2nd, Lu P, Blesch A, et al. IGF-I gene delivery promotes corticospinal neuronal survival but not regeneration after adult CNS injury. Exp Neurol 2009;215(1):53–9.

56. Sendtner M, Kreutzberg GW, Thoenen H. Ciliary neurotrophic factor prevents the degeneration of motor neurons after axotomy. Nature 1990; 345(6274):440–1.

57. Sendtner M, Holtmann B, Kolbeck R, et al. Brain-derived neurotrophic factor prevents the death of motoneurons in newborn rats after nerve section. Nature 1992;360(6406):757–9.

58. Conta Steencken AC, Smirnov I, Stelzner DJ. Cell survival or cell death: differential vulnerability of long descending and thoracic propriospinal neurons to low thoracic axotomy in the adult rat. Neuroscience 2011;194:359–71.

59. McBride RL, Feringa ER, Garver MK, et al. Prelabeled red nucleus and sensorimotor cortex neurons of the rat survive 10 and 20 weeks after spinal cord transection. J Neuropathol Exp Neurol 1989;48(5): 568–76.

60. Merline M, Kalil K. Cell death of corticospinal neurons is induced by axotomy before but not after innervation of spinal targets. J Comp Neurol 1990; 296(3):506–16.

61. Tran NM, Shekhar K, Whitney IE, et al. Single-cell profiles of retinal ganglion cells differing in resilience to injury reveal neuroprotective genes. Neuron 2019; 104(6):1039–55.e12.

62. Shekhar K, Lapan SW, Whitney IE, et al. Comprehensive classification of retinal bipolar neurons by single-cell transcriptomics. Cell 2016;166(5): 1308–23.e30.

63. Haring M, Zeisel A, Hochgerner H, et al. Neuronal atlas of the dorsal horn defines its architecture and links sensory input to transcriptional cell types. Nat Neurosci 2018;21(6):869–80.

64. Sathyamurthy A, Johnson KR, Matson KJE, et al. Massively parallel single nucleus transcriptional profiling defines spinal cord neurons and their activity during behavior. Cell Rep 2018;22(8):2216–25.

65. Zeisel A, Hochgerner H, Lonnerberg P, et al. Molecular architecture of the mouse nervous system. Cell 2018;174(4):999–1014.e22.

66. Skinnider MA, Squair JW, Kathe C, et al. Cell type prioritization in single-cell data. Nat Biotechnol 2020. https://doi.org/10.1038/s41587-020-0605-1.

67. Yin Y, Cui Q, Li Y, et al. Macrophage-derived factors stimulate optic nerve regeneration. J Neurosci 2003; 23(6):2284–93.

68. Aguayo AJ, Rasminsky M, Bray GM, et al. Degenerative and regenerative responses of injured neurons in the central nervous system of adult mammals. Philos Trans R Soc Lond B Biol Sci 1991; 331(1261):337–43.

69. Goldberg JL, Espinosa JS, Xu Y, et al. Retinal ganglion cells do not extend axons by default: promotion by neurotrophic signaling and electrical activity. Neuron 2002;33(5):689–702.

70. Goldberg JL, Barres BA. The relationship between neuronal survival and regeneration. Annu Rev Neurosci 2000;23:579–612.

71. Shen S, Wiemelt AP, McMorris FA, et al. Retinal ganglion cells lose trophic responsiveness after axotomy. Neuron 1999;23(2):285–95.

72. Lucius R, Gallinat S, Rosenstiel P, et al. The angiotensin II type 2 (AT2) receptor promotes axonal regeneration in the optic nerve of adult rats. J Exp Med 1998;188(4):661–70.

73. Alto LT, Havton LA, Conner JM, et al. Chemotropic guidance facilitates axonal regeneration and synapse formation after spinal cord injury. Nat Neurosci 2009;12(9):1106–13.

74. Deng L-X, Deng P, Ruan Y, et al. A novel growth-promoting pathway formed by GDNF-overexpressing Schwann cells promotes propriospinal axonal regeneration, synapse formation, and partial recovery of function after spinal cord injury. J Neurosci 2013;33(13): 5655–67.

75. He Z, Jin Y. Intrinsic control of axon regeneration. Neuron 2016;90(3):437–51.

76. Mahar M, Cavalli V. Intrinsic mechanisms of neuronal axon regeneration. Nat Rev Neurosci 2018;19(6): 323–37.

77. Liu K, Tedeschi A, Park KK, et al. Neuronal intrinsic mechanisms of axon regeneration. Annu Rev Neurosci 2011;34:131–52.

78. Park KK, Liu K, Hu Y, et al. Promoting axon regeneration in the adult CNS by modulation of the PTEN/mTOR pathway. Science 2008;322(5903):963–6.

79. Smith PD, Sun F, Park KK, et al. SOCS3 deletion promotes optic nerve regeneration in vivo. Neuron 2009;64(5):617–23.

80. Belin S, Nawabi H, Wang C, et al. Injury-induced decline of intrinsic regenerative ability revealed by quantitative proteomics. Neuron 2015;86(4): 1000–14.

81. Nawabi H, Belin S, Cartoni R, et al. Doublecortin-like kinases promote neuronal survival and induce growth cone reformation via distinct mechanisms. Neuron 2015;88. https://doi.org/10.1016/j.neuron. 2015.10.005.

82. Moore DL, Blackmore MG, Hu Y, et al. KLF family members regulate intrinsic axon regeneration ability. Science 2009;326(5950):298–301.

83. Norsworthy MW, Bei F, Kawaguchi R, et al. Sox11 expression promotes regeneration of some retinal ganglion cell types but kills others. Neuron 2017; 94(6):1112–20.e4.

84. Fenrich KK, Rose PK. Spinal interneuron axons spontaneously regenerate after spinal cord injury in the adult feline. J Neurosci 2009;29(39): 12145–58.

85. Lu P, Wang Y, Graham L, et al. Long-distance growth and connectivity of neural stem cells after severe spinal cord injury. Cell 2012;150(6):1264–73.

86. Kadoya K, Lu P, Nguyen K, et al. Spinal cord reconstitution with homologous neural grafts enables robust corticospinal regeneration. Nat Med 2016; 22(5):479–87.

87. Poplawski GHD, Kawaguchi R, Van Niekerk E, et al. Injured adult neurons regress to an embryonic transcriptional growth state. Nature 2020;581(7806): 77–82.

Brain-Computer Interface, Neuromodulation, and Neurorehabilitation Strategies for Spinal Cord Injury

Iahn Cajigas, MD, PhD*, Aditya Vedantam, MD

KEYWORDS

- Neuromodulation • Neural interfaces • Brain-computer interfaces • Neurorehabilitation
- Neural plasticity

KEY POINTS

- There has been significant progress in the use of brain-computer interface, neuromodulation, and neurorehabilitation strategies to help restore function after spinal cord injury (SCI).
- Many brain-computer (neural bypass) interfaces aim to translate cortical signals into peripheral motor responses, in effect bypassing spinal cord lesions.
- Neuromodulation strategies aim to recruit residual functional spinal/supraspinal circuits and/or potentiate the formation of new functional connections within the nervous system.
- Neurorehabilitation strategies have been shown improve neurologic function in patients with incomplete SCI and lead to improvement in cardiovascular and metabolic functions that are associated with improved quality of life.

INTRODUCTION

Over the past several decades, survival rates following acute spinal cord injury (SCI) have increased substantially, paralleled by a similar increase in life expectancy,[1,2] making restoration of function a central focus of current research in order to maximize community independence. Many different therapeutic modalities have been explored to improve outcomes in people with chronic SCI. This article reviews some of the recent progress in brain-computer interfacing, neuromodulation, and neurorehabilitation for functional restoration in patients with SCI (**Fig. 1**).

BRAIN-COMPUTER INTERFACING

Neural interface research has been strongly motivated by the need to restore communication and control to more than 5.4 million individuals in the United States with various neurologic disorders and diseases of the central and peripheral nervous system such as stroke (33.7%), SCI (27.3%), and multiple sclerosis (18.6%) resulting in paralysis.[3–8] The long-term use of rehabilitative neuroprosthetics could significantly improve the quality of life of paralyzed individuals with technology to reanimate nonfunctional limbs, replace missing limbs, and enable new modes of direct neural communication.[3,6]

Over the last 20 years, there has been a surge in the number of successful applications of brain-computer interfaces (BCIs) for upper extremity control involving reaching and grasping.[9–14] However, current implantable neural bypass systems for tetraplegia require patients to be constantly tethered to an external power source and recording hardware, limiting their application to a laboratory setting.[9,11,15] Further, decoding algorithms generally rely on single-neuron

Department of Neurosurgery, University of Miami, 1095 Northwest 14th Terrace (D4-6), Miami, FL 33136, USA
* Corresponding author.
E-mail address: icajigas@med.miami.edu
Twitter: @iahncajigas (I.C.)

Neurosurg Clin N Am 32 (2021) 407–417
https://doi.org/10.1016/j.nec.2021.03.012
1042-3680/21/© 2021 Elsevier Inc. All rights reserved.

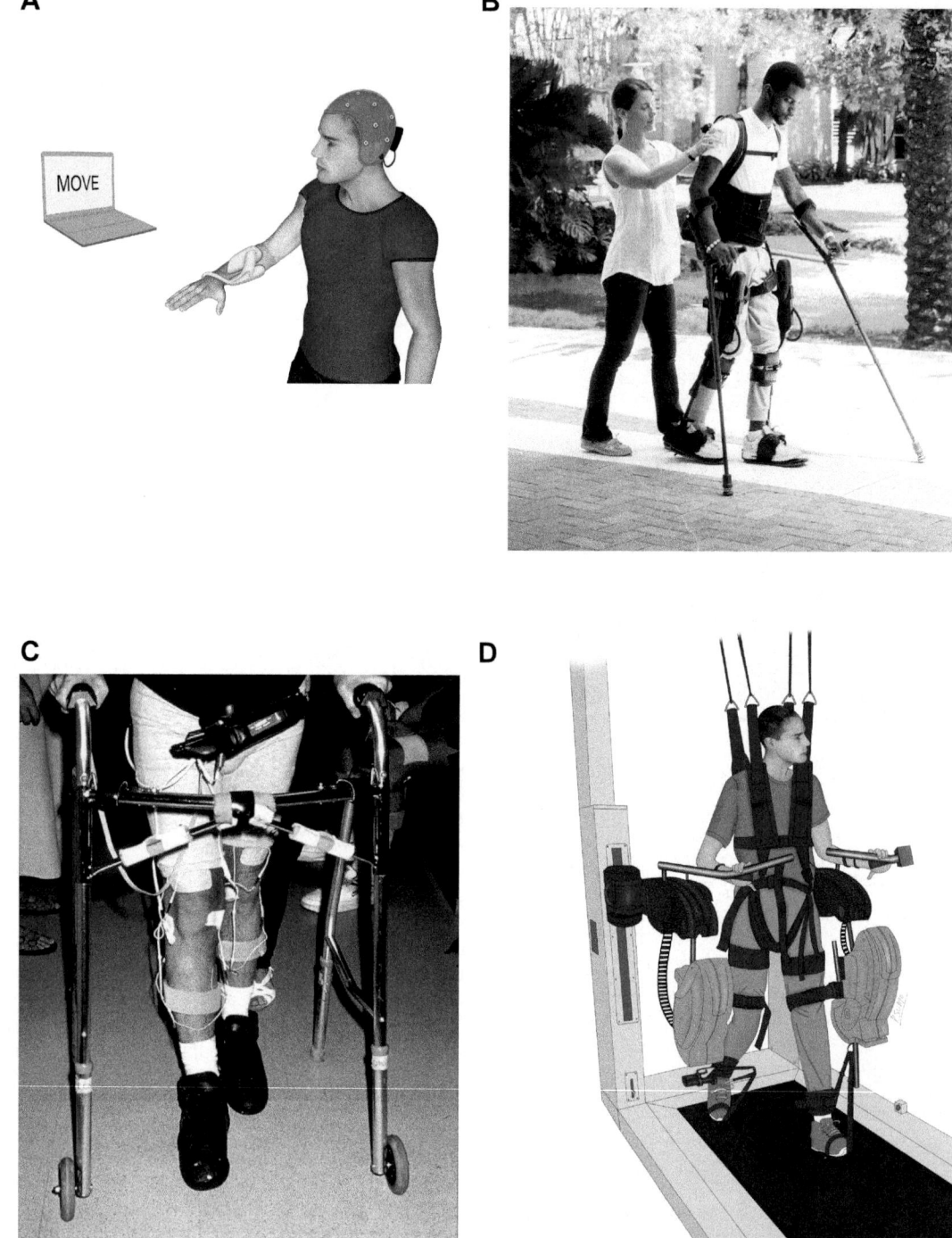

Fig. 1. (*A*) A brain-computer interface driven by event-related desynchronizations detected on scalp electroencephalogram when a patient with spinal cord injury with cervical quadriplegia thinks about moving the dominant upper extremity and is used to trigger functional electrical stimulation of the dominant right upper extremity, as described by Gant and colleagues.[23] (*B*) Patient with thoracic SCI walking with the assistance of an exoskeleton. (*C*) A patient with incomplete SCI ambulates with the assistance of a walker using functional electrical stimulation of the lower extremity muscles. (*D*) Robotic-assisted weight-supported treadmill training being using in a patient with SCI to facilitate high-intensity training. (Photo in B courtesy of Dr. Jennifer Maher, Dr. Mark S. Nash, and Robert Camarena at the Miami Project to Cure Paralysis.)

activity,[10,12,14] the recording quality of which degrades over time in animals and humans.[16] Motivated by this observation, studies have sought to develop algorithms that rely on electroencephalography (EEG) signals recorded noninvasively from the scalp.[17–20] However, these signals suffer from low signal-to-noise ratio and are therefore prone to contamination from artifact.

Further studies have relied on more stable electrocorticography (ECoG) signals recorded from the brain surface.[19] These latter attempts have thus far been limited to temporary implantations because of the clinical indications for ECoG (eg, seizure mapping).[19] Successive continuous movement of the hands was first noticed by Jasper and Penfield[21] in 1949 to block beta rhythm in the precentral and postcentral hand area measured by ECoG.[21] Interestingly, these beta-rhythm reductions, called event-related desynchronizations (ERDs), are also observed during imagined movements of the limb. Recently, a fully implanted ECoG-based BCI triggered by ERDs successfully allowed a locked-in patient with amyotrophic lateral sclerosis (ALS) to communicate through typing.[22] Therefore, it is not surprising that ERDs and other frequency characteristics of the EEG and ECoG are at the forefront of current research for a variety of end-organ uses from controlling a cursor on a computer screen[18] to moving paralyzed muscles.[23]

Surface activity recorded from the sensorimotor cortex of the upper limb with bilateral wireless 64-channel epidural electrodes has been used to promote movement in a patient with C4 American Spinal Injury Association Impairment Scale (AIS) A SCI. An adaptive decoding algorithm was used to send commands to either a virtual avatar or an exoskeleton during a 24-month trial. Over the duration of the trial, the subject was able to control activation of a 4-limb neuroprosthetic exoskeleton (up to 8 degrees of freedom) simultaneously without recalibration for up to 7 weeks.[24] Continued improvements in computational power governing implantable circuits suggest the possibility of even more sophisticated BCIs emerging in the short term.

Neuromodulation After Spinal Cord Injury

Neuromodulation makes use of electrical stimulation to modify neuronal activity in the central and peripheral nervous systems. The goal of neuromodulatory strategies in SCI are to recruit residual functional spinal/supraspinal circuits to improve function, and/or to potentiate formation of new neuronal connections within the nervous system to replace damaged networks. Improved

understanding of spinal cord circuits in animals has led to translation of neuromodulation to assist neurologic rehabilitation after human SCI.

Scientific basis

The central nervous system shows both structural and functional changes after injury. Animal studies show spontaneous formation of new neural circuits in spared neural fibers after SCI.[25–27] Preservation of corticospinal connections after incomplete cervical SCI has been shown to be essential to spontaneous motor recovery.[28] Cortical input to brainstem reticulospinal axons also contributes to recovery of hindlimb function after incomplete SCI.[25] Both maladaptive (ie, increased spasticity, gliosis) and positive functional (ie, migrations of neurons across site of injury) changes occur in intraspinal neural circuits and motor neurons after SCI, further highlighting neuroplasticity along the neuroaxis after injury.[26] Together, this information provides evidence for innate adaptations of the central nervous system after SCI.

Deep brain stimulation, spinal cord stimulation, epidural electrical stimulation, functional electrical stimulation, and peripheral nerve stimulation are types of neuromodulation that have been explored in the context of SCI. These modalities stimulate descending neuronal fibers, spared motor neuron, and interneuron circuits.[29] Repeated stimulation of these targets can produce functional reorganization, which can lead to regeneration and new neuronal connections.[30] Activity-based neuroplasticity, which forms the basis of physical rehabilitation, can be paired with electric neuromodulation to enhance gains in motor function.[31,32] The induction of neuroplasticity by combining these 2 complimentary techniques has been the most successful approach in spinal cord neuromodulation. There is mounting evidence that multimodal techniques using BCI, neuromodulation, and neurorehabilitation may have augmented effects compared with their individual application.[33]

Epidural spinal cord stimulation

Epidural spinal cord stimulation (SCS) using surgically implanted electrodes in the posterior epidural space was initially used to treat chronic pain. Early investigators expanded the use of epidural SCS and noted considerable improvements in spasticity, bladder function, and motor function in patients with multiple sclerosis.[34] Studies investigating epidural SCS in subjects with SCI found that stimulation below the level of injury produced improvements in spasticity, and in some cases motor recovery,[35,36] to a greater degree than stimulation above the level of injury.[31,37] Epidural SCS in the conus region (L1-L2) has been shown to control severe spasticity in patients with chronic SCI.[38] Those with incomplete SCI may benefit more than those with complete SCI.[37] Motor unit activity has been seen to increase in some patients undergoing epidural SCS, suggesting that stimulation may improve motor function in addition to reducing spasticity.[39]

Mechanism of action

The primary intrathecal target in lumbar SCS is the posterior sensory roots with large and medium fiber afferents arising from the lower limbs and ascending primarily in the dorsal columns.[40,41] Proprioceptive afferents and muscle spindle feedback are essential for locomotor recovery after SCI.[27,42] Lumbar epidural SCS activates these afferents in addition to firing spinal interneurons and motor neurons via intraspinal monosynaptic and polysynaptic circuits.[43] In incomplete SCI, it is also thought that stimulation of the posterior columns creates orthodromic signals that affect brainstem control (via reticulospinal pathways) of the lumbar intraspinal circuits. These mechanisms are postulated to contribute to increased spontaneous motor activity and improved voluntary control.

The effect of epidural SCS on complex lower limb movement is amplified by increasing the state of excitability of the intraspinal circuit.[35] Intensive motor training increases the excitability of the lumbar motor circuits, and has been shown to improve functional intraspinal connections.[44] In a rat SCI model, lumbar epidural SCS complemented with motor training led to improved hindlimb motor function via activation of previously silent axonal projections across the lesion.[45] Importantly, active initiation of hindlimb movement by the injured animal is critical to neuroplasticity induced by lumbar epidural SCS.[46] Animal SCI models have been used to better understand the configuration of lumbar epidural SCS required to induce gait and locomotor motion.[46] Real-time electromyography recordings from leg muscles during gait and stimulation have been used to further refine lumbar epidural SCS from tonic stimulation to specific spatiotemporal activations, facilitating more rapid improvement in locomotion after injury.[47] Spatiotemporal lumbar epidural SCS can be coupled with intracranial microelectrode arrays to decode motor cortex signals responsible for gait. The culmination of these experiments was the demonstration of a wireless system that decodes intracranial motor cortex signals, bypasses the lesion, and produces specific epidural lumbar SCS to restore locomotion after primate SCI.[48]

A newer, reversible, and painless paraplegia model has recently been developed with the hope of making device development in nonhuman primates more accessible to other laboratories hoping to show efficacy of certain bypass BCI devices in primates without needing to induce permanent SCI.[49]

Clinical Efficacy

Improved voluntary motor activity after lumbar epidural SCS was first reported in a single patient with a chronic motor complete T1 SCI. The patient underwent surgical placement of a 16-electrode array in the conus region. Tonic epidural stimulation, combined with intensive locomotor training, was able to induce voluntary leg movements and help with weight bearing, standing, and stepping.[36] The same team repeated this experiment in 3 other patients with chronic SCI and showed that neuromodulation of lumbosacral networks was able to restore voluntary leg movements. Intensive rehabilitation further improved the gains observed with epidural SCS, allowing patients with SCI to stand independently with full weight bearing for short periods of time.[35] These studies provided a remarkable demonstration of motor reactivation in chronically paralyzed limbs after SCI.

Epidural SCS also produces improvements in other neurologic deficits, such as voluntary control of bladder function,[50] normalization of blood pressure,[51] improved sexual function,[52] and body composition[53] in patients with SCI. Current evidence supports the theory that patients most likely to show improvement from epidural conus stimulation have an incomplete, or discomplete,[54] SCI (ie, clinically complete but with evidence of anatomically intact fibers spanning the lesion) and an intact conus medullaris, because attempts to apply this treatment to patients without these features have been less successful.[55]

In contrast with tonic stimulation, spatiotemporal epidural stimulation can produce specific leg movements associated with gait. This technique involves identifying areas in the spinal cord that are active during a specific gait phase. A closed-loop system of inertial sensors identifies the phase of gait of the participant and then synchronizes the electrical impulses to the corresponding muscle groups. This type of simulation seems to be superior to continuous epidural SCS and enables over-ground ambulation.[56] When combined with a rehabilitation program, SCI participants show substantial improvements in walking and voluntary leg movements with and without epidural SCS.[57] The development of closed-loop systems for spatiotemporal epidural SCS is a step toward expanding the use of neuromodulation in a home environment for patients with SCI.

Transcutaneous spinal cord stimulation

Transcutaneous stimulation of the spinal cord is being explored as a minimally invasive technique to activate local spinal cord circuitry. Electrodes are placed on the skin, and direct current stimulation is used for neuromodulation. Stimulation protocols include both biphasic and monophasic currents with high-frequency pulses. Most studies use high-intensity currents that near the threshold tolerated by participants.[58] Similar to epidural SCS, transcutaneous SCS targets the proprioceptive pathways via the posterior roots.[59] Transcutaneous SCS can modulate both upper and lower limb function. Transcutaneous SCS combined with training can produce sustained gains in bilateral hand function after chronic incomplete cervical SCI[60] and has been shown to produce volitional stepping in the lower limbs.[61] Most case reports and small series using this technique have studied participants with incomplete SCI, and have included a training paradigm in addition to transcutaneous SCS.[58] Transcutaneous SCS produces increased electromyographic activity in the corresponding muscles, and enhances voluntary motor control and trunk stability.[61,62] Commercially available cutaneous electrodes are easier to set up and less inexpensive than epidural SCS. Limitations of transcutaneous SCS include stimulation-induced sensory side effects as well as the lack of fine spatiotemporal stimulation to activate specific muscle groups.

Transcranial magnetic stimulation

Studies in subjects with clinically complete SCI have shown evidence of spared anatomic and functional connections across the lesion.[63,64] In 1 report, more than half the subjects with AIS A and B SCI showed preservation of volitional electromyographic responses in muscles innervated below the neurologic level of injury.[65] A small proportion of patients continued to show neurologic improvement after complete SCI even at 1 to 5 years after the injury.[66] Transcranial stimulation to induce motor movement is predicated on preservation of supraspinal connections across the level of SCI. Transcranial magnetic stimulation (TMS) generates electrical responses in the cortex using magnetic fields, which is less painful than electrical stimulation. Direct activation of corticospinal neurons as well as indirect synaptic stimulation of these neurons produce signals along the corticospinal tract.[67] Repetitive TMS over the motor cortex can produce motor movement via this cortical activation. These effects depend on duration of the magnetic stimulation, direction of the field, and cortical excitability.[68–70] Voluntary task-based motor activity increases cortical excitability and can augment cortical stimulation via TMS.[70] In patients with SCI, TMS impulses can improve grasp strength when combined with task-based hand activity.[71] When paired with peripheral nerve stimulation, timed TMS modulates synaptic transmission between corticospinal fibers and anterior horn cells. This process has been shown to augment hand function in tetraplegic patients undergoing TMS.[72] Other studies have shown that TMS improves ambulation in patients with incomplete SCI when combined with locomotor training,[73] pointing to the positive effect of TMS on corticospinal plasticity. TMS is a promising adjunct to rehabilitation and training protocols.

Challenges and future areas of research

Despite promising results, neuromodulation for SCI faces several challenges.[74] Some of the approaches, such as epidural SCS, include totally implantable components and can be used by participants in their home environments. However, technologies that access supraspinal circuits, such as TMS, require nonportable, specialized, and costly external machines along with user expertise. The clinical translation of wireless cortical implants that communicate with lumbar epidural electrodes[75] will further push the boundaries of accessible neuromodulation for patients with SCI. At this time, the mechanism of action of these technologies has been incompletely elucidated, and a better understanding of spinal neuroplasticity is necessary to optimize stimulation paradigms. As described earlier, most studies are limited to small case series and case reports; large-scale clinical trials are awaited to validate the early positive results. In addition, long-term durability and cost will need to be addressed to maximize access and adoption of this technique for patients with SCI.

NEUROREHABILITATION

The most common neurorehabilitation interventions for SCI include functional electrical stimulation, high-intensity repetitive movement training, use of robotic exoskeletons to assist with physical therapy, and combination therapies that leverage simultaneous neuromodulation and intense physical therapy.[76] Although a detailed description of each of the neurorehabilitation approaches is outside the scope of this article, a few of the most widely used techniques are reviewed.

FUNCTIONAL ELECTRICAL STIMULATION

Functional electrical stimulation (FES) consists of the application of small electrodes to paralyzed muscles through which electrical pulses are delivered to help restore or improve function. In patients with complete or incomplete SCI, there is now proof of FES-induced activation of central pattern generators within the spinal cord responsible for locomotion. Increased stepping responses have been observed in response to FES.[36,77,78] In addition, some patients regularly treated with FES have shown improved AIS motor and sensory scores[79] and decreased spasticity.[80]

In addition to the neurophysiologic changes observed with FES, overall health measures have also shown significant positive improvements. These improvements tend to be more immediate and can significantly improve quality of life.[81] The most well-studied effect of FES is the subsequent improvement in muscle size, strength, and composition with overall improved oxidative capacity[81] and fatigue resistance.[82] Recovery of lost bone mass, particularly in the lower extremities, has also been reported with FES.[83] Moreover, improvements in cardiovascular conditioning and metabolic function (ie, decreased insulin resistance[84] and decreased adipose tissue[85]) have also been shown in patients with SCI.

HIGH-INTENSITY, HIGH-VOLUME TARGETED TRAINING

Recent SCI rehabilitation has concentrated on the delivery of high-intensity, high-volume, repetitive rehabilitative exercises, providing clinical improvements to both patients with complete SCI and patients with incomplete SCI.[86] Approaches such as activity-based restorative therapy were developed from the understanding that motor activation could be achieved with intensive training following motor injury or complete transection.[87–93] This work is based on the theory that locomotion after SCI could be preserved by repetitive training in tandem with the simulation of central pattern generators (CPGs), ambulatory motor reflex pathways operating without brain input below the level of SCI.[86,92,93] Studies by Grillner and others have explored the underlying function of CPGs, showing that spinalized cats can be conditioned to stand, attain full hindlimb weight-bearing strength, and achieve locomotion at varying speeds on a treadmill with intensive physical training.[89,93,94] Weight-bearing activity is an important component of post-SCI rehabilitation, because Harkema and coworkers have shown treadmill activity to increase spontaneous hip

extensor activity following injury.[92,94] However, patients with motor complete SCI are a more complex entity and have so far proved refractory to clinical benefit from intensive locomotor training.[92,95,96]

EXOSKELETON USE IN SPINAL CORD INJURY

Exoskeleton use in acute rehabilitation and for long-term activities of daily living (ADL) represents a novel approach to the complex biological processes of central nervous system regeneration and repair that have curbed progress in many areas of SCI treatment. Accompanying the rapid process of muscle atrophy following SCI, especially in the context of complete SCI, are several cellular mechanisms that remain poorly understood.[97,98] As such, increased exertional effort required by patients with SCI for even small tasks, although extremely beneficial in the acute SCI period, ultimately limits rehabilitation efforts, expends significant levels of energy with or without an orthosis or wheelchair, and can significantly limit a patient's ADLs.[99] Exoskeletons have emerged as a way to address some of the limitations of body weight–supported treadmill training, which is frequently used to restore the ability to walk after SCI but is significantly limited by fatigue of patients and therapists.[100] The use of passive or actively powered robotic exoskeletons increases efficiency of work by supporting weakened stabilizer muscles, increasing sustainable workloads, and decreasing energy use by both patient and therapist. Actively powered robotic exoskeletons use an external battery source, support joints at risk for injury, are ergonomic, and are becoming more efficient in design.[101]

More recently, Grasmücke and coworkers implemented a Hybrid Assistive Limb Exoskeleton (Hal, Cyberdyne Inc, Japan), which uses electromyographic stimuli from a wearer with incomplete SCI to serve as an impulse for gait and limb assistance within the powered exoskeleton. They report through their experiences that motivated patients can be trained effectively using this device to improve ADLs.[102,103] Although neither the Hal or any other exoskeleton is a permanent substitute for daily ambulation yet, these incremental advancements in exoskeleton technology and efficiency are gradually improving the lives of patients with SCI. There are currently numerous treadmill-based and fully mobile exoskeletons being tested in clinical trials that may alter how patients with chronic SCI receive therapy in and out of the hospital in the near future. Although there are nuances to each exoskeleton and study protocol, the results of these trials generally support the idea that exoskeletons help patients improve cardiopulmonary function and muscle physiology, and potentially improve walking performance.[100,104,105]

SUMMARY

The drive to restore motor function and independence in patients with SCI has driven numerous developments within neuromodulation, neurorehabilitation, and brain-computer interfacing. There is mounting evidence that combinations of each of these techniques may yield superior outcomes compared with when each is used separately. Clinical experience on a large scale will be required to determine the optimal combinations of the distinct interventions that yield the best outcome, and this is likely to depend significantly on the level of residual neural function for each patient. However, the continued improvements that have been shown in chronic SCI, previously thought impossible, raise the possibility of significant improvements in the function and quality of life of individuals affected with SCI.

CLINICS CARE POINTS

- BCI, neuromodulation, and neurorehabilitation approaches have been developed to maximize motor function and restore functional independence after SCI.
- Even in the absence of improvements in motor function, modest improvements in cardiovascular and metabolic function achieved via neurorehabilitation can yield a significant improvement in quality of life.
- Current clinical applications of these techniques typically leverage combinations of multiple modalities because these have shown the most promising results.

ACKNOWLEDGEMENT

Iahn Cajigas IC was supported in part by NIH R25NS108937-02.

DISCLOSURE

The authors have nothing to disclose.

REFERENCES

1. Barbeau H, Nadeau S, Garneau C. Physical determinants, emerging concepts, and training approaches in gait of individuals with spinal cord injury. J Neurotrauma 2006;23(3–4):571–85.
2. Nobunaga AI, Go BK, Karunas RB. Recent demographic and injury trends in people served by the Model Spinal Cord Injury Care Systems. Arch Phys Med Rehabil 1999;80(11):1372–82.
3. Anderson KD. Consideration of user priorities when developing neural prosthetics. J Neural Eng 2009;6(5):055003.
4. Aravamudhan S, Bellamkonda RV. Toward a convergence of regenerative medicine, rehabilitation, and neuroprosthetics. J Neurotrauma 2011;28(11):2329–47.
5. Armour BS, Courtney-Long EA, Fox MH, et al. Prevalence and causes of Paralysis-United States, 2013. Am J Public Health 2016;106(10):1855–7.
6. Nicolelis MA. Brain-machine interfaces to restore motor function and probe neural circuits. Nat Rev Neurosci 2003;4(5):417–22.
7. Wolpaw JR, Birbaumer N, Heetderks WJ, et al. Brain-computer interface technology: a review of the first international meeting. IEEE Trans Rehabil Eng 2000;8(2):164–73.
8. Wolpaw JR, Birbaumer N, McFarland DJ, et al. Brain-computer interfaces for communication and control. Clin Neurophysiol 2002;113(6):767–91.
9. Ajiboye AB, Willett FR, Young DR, et al. Restoration of reaching and grasping movements through brain-controlled muscle stimulation in a person with tetraplegia: a proof-of-concept demonstration. Lancet 2017;389(10081):1821–30.
10. Chapin JK, Moxon KA, Markowitz RS, et al. Real-time control of a robot arm using simultaneously recorded neurons in the motor cortex. Nat Neurosci 1999;2(7):664–70.
11. Collinger JL, Wodlinger B, Downey JE, et al. High-performance neuroprosthetic control by an individual with tetraplegia. Lancet 2013;381(9866):557–64.
12. Hochberg LR, Bacher D, Jarosiewicz B, et al. Reach and grasp by people with tetraplegia using a neurally controlled robotic arm. Nature 2012;485(7398):372–5.
13. Hochberg LR, Serruya MD, Friehs GM, et al. Neuronal ensemble control of prosthetic devices by a human with tetraplegia. Nature 2006;442(7099):164–71.
14. Velliste M, Perel S, Spalding MC, et al. Cortical control of a prosthetic arm for self-feeding. Nature 2008;453(7198):1098–101.
15. Bouton CE, Shaikhouni A, Annetta NV, et al. Restoring cortical control of functional movement in a human with quadriplegia. Nature 2016;533(7602):247–50.
16. Gunasekera B, Saxena T, Bellamkonda R, et al. Intracortical recording interfaces: current challenges to chronic recording function. ACS Chem Neurosci 2015;6(1):68–83.

17. Heasman JM, Scott TR, Kirkup L, et al. Control of a hand grasp neuroprosthesis using an electroencephalogram-triggered switch: demonstration of improvements in performance using wavepacket analysis. Med Biol Eng Comput 2002;40(5):588–93.

18. Wolpaw JR, McFarland DJ. Control of a two-dimensional movement signal by a noninvasive brain-computer interface in humans. Proc Natl Acad Sci U S A 2004;101(51):17849–54.

19. Wang W, Collinger JL, Degenhart AD, et al. An electrocorticographic brain interface in an individual with tetraplegia. PLoS One 2013;8(2):e55344.

20. Meng J, Edelman BJ, Olsoe J, et al. A study of the effects of electrode number and decoding algorithm on online eeg-based bci behavioral performance. Front Neurosci 2018;12:227.

21. Jasper H, Penfield W. Electrocorticograms in man: effect of voluntary movement upon the electrical activity of the precentral gyrus. Archiv für Psychiatrie und Nervenkrankheiten 1949;183(1–2):163–74.

22. Vansteensel MJ, Pels EGM, Bleichner MG, et al. Fully implanted brain-computer interface in a locked-in patient with ALS. N Engl J Med 2016;375(21):2060–6.

23. Gant K, Guerra S, Zimmerman L, et al. EEG-controlled functional electrical stimulation for hand opening and closing in chronic complete cervical spinal cord injury. Biomed Phys Eng Express 2018;4(6):065005.

24. Benabid AL, Costecalde T, Eliseyev A, et al. An exoskeleton controlled by an epidural wireless brain-machine interface in a tetraplegic patient: a proof-of-concept demonstration. Lancet Neurol 2019;18(12):1112–22.

25. Asboth L, Friedli L, Beauparlant J, et al. Cortico-reticulo-spinal circuit reorganization enables functional recovery after severe spinal cord contusion. Nat Neurosci 2018;21(4):576–88.

26. Bellardita C, Caggiano V, Leiras R, et al. Spatiotemporal correlation of spinal network dynamics underlying spasms in chronic spinalized mice. Elife 2017;6:e23011.

27. Takeoka A, Vollenweider I, Courtine G, et al. Muscle spindle feedback directs locomotor recovery and circuit reorganization after spinal cord injury. Cell 2014;159(7):1626–39.

28. Hilton BJ, Anenberg E, Harrison TC, et al. Re-establishment of cortical motor output maps and spontaneous functional recovery via spared dorsolaterally projecting corticospinal neurons after dorsal column spinal cord injury in adult mice. J Neurosci 2016;36(14):4080–92.

29. Courtine G, Sofroniew MV. Spinal cord repair: advances in biology and technology. Nat Med 2019;25(6):898–908.

30. Gill ML, Grahn PJ, Calvert JS, et al. Neuromodulation of lumbosacral spinal networks enables independent stepping after complete paraplegia. Nat Med 2018;24(11):1677–82.

31. Krucoff MO, Miller JP, Saxena T, et al. Toward functional restoration of the central nervous system: a review of translational neuroscience principles. Neurosurgery 2019;84(1):30–40.

32. Rejc E, Angeli CA, Atkinson D, et al. Motor recovery after activity-based training with spinal cord epidural stimulation in a chronic motor complete paraplegic. Sci Rep 2017;7(1):13476.

33. Krucoff MO, Rahimpour S, Slutzky MW, et al. Enhancing nervous system recovery through neurobiologics, neural interface training, and neurorehabilitation. Front Neurosci 2016;10:584.

34. Eisdorfer JT, Smit RD, Keefe KM, et al. Epidural electrical stimulation: a review of plasticity mechanisms that are hypothesized to underlie enhanced recovery from spinal cord injury with stimulation. Front Mol Neurosci 2020;13:163.

35. Angeli CA, Edgerton VR, Gerasimenko YP, et al. Altering spinal cord excitability enables voluntary movements after chronic complete paralysis in humans. Brain 2014;137(Pt 5):1394–409.

36. Harkema S, Gerasimenko Y, Hodes J, et al. Effect of epidural stimulation of the lumbosacral spinal cord on voluntary movement, standing, and assisted stepping after motor complete paraplegia: a case study. Lancet 2011;377(9781):1938–47.

37. Dimitrijevic MM, Dimitrijevic MR, Illis LS, et al. Spinal cord stimulation for the control of spasticity in patients with chronic spinal cord injury: I. Clinical observations. Cent Nerv Syst Trauma 1986;3(2):129–44.

38. Pinter MM, Gerstenbrand F, Dimitrijevic MR. Epidural electrical stimulation of posterior structures of the human lumbosacral cord: 3. Control of spasticity. Spinal Cord 2000;38(9):524–31.

39. Dimitrijevic MR, Illis LS, Nakajima K, et al. Spinal cord stimulation for the control of spasticity in patients with chronic spinal cord injury: II. Neurophysiologic observations. Cent Nerv Syst Trauma 1986;3(2):145–52.

40. Capogrosso M, Wenger N, Raspopovic S, et al. A computational model for epidural electrical stimulation of spinal sensorimotor circuits. J Neurosci 2013;33(49):19326–40.

41. Courtine G, Gerasimenko Y, van den Brand R, et al. Transformation of nonfunctional spinal circuits into functional states after the loss of brain input. Nat Neurosci 2009;12(10):1333–42.

42. Takeoka A, Arber S. Functional local proprioceptive feedback circuits initiate and maintain locomotor recovery after spinal cord injury. Cell Rep 2019;27(1):71–85.e73.

43. Minassian K, Persy I, Rattay F, et al. Human lumbar cord circuitries can be activated by extrinsic tonic input to generate locomotor-like activity. Hum Mov Sci 2007;26(2):275–95.

44. Wang H, Liu NK, Zhang YP, et al. Treadmill training induced lumbar motoneuron dendritic plasticity and behavior recovery in adult rats after a thoracic contusive spinal cord injury. Exp Neurol 2015;271:368–78.

45. van den Brand R, Heutschi J, Barraud Q, et al. Restoring voluntary control of locomotion after paralyzing spinal cord injury. Science 2012; 336(6085):1182–5.

46. Capogrosso M, Wagner FB, Gandar J, et al. Configuration of electrical spinal cord stimulation through real-time processing of gait kinematics. Nat Protoc 2018;13(9):2031–61.

47. Wenger N, Moraud EM, Gandar J, et al. Spatiotemporal neuromodulation therapies engaging muscle synergies improve motor control after spinal cord injury. Nat Med 2016;22(2):138–45.

48. Bonizzato M, Pidpruzhnykova G, DiGiovanna J, et al. Brain-controlled modulation of spinal circuits improves recovery from spinal cord injury. Nat Commun 2018;9(1):3015.

49. Krucoff MO, Zhuang K, MacLeod D, et al. A novel paraplegia model in awake behaving macaques. J Neurophysiol 2017;118(3):1800–8.

50. Herrity AN, Williams CS, Angeli CA, et al. Lumbosacral spinal cord epidural stimulation improves voiding function after human spinal cord injury. Sci Rep 2018;8(1):8688.

51. Harkema SJ, Wang S, Angeli CA, et al. Normalization of blood pressure with spinal cord epidural stimulation after severe spinal cord injury. Front Hum Neurosci 2018;12:83.

52. Darrow D, Balser D, Netoff TI, et al. Epidural spinal cord stimulation facilitates immediate restoration of dormant motor and autonomic supraspinal pathways after chronic neurologically complete spinal cord injury. J Neurotrauma 2019;36(15):2325–36.

53. Terson de Paleville DGL, Harkema SJ, Angeli CA. Epidural stimulation with locomotor training improves body composition in individuals with cervical or upper thoracic motor complete spinal cord injury: a series of case studies. J Spinal Cord Med 2019;42(1):32–8.

54. Dimitrijevic MR. Neurophysiology in spinal cord injury. Paraplegia 1987;25(3):205–8.

55. Krucoff MO, Gramer R, Lott D, et al. Spinal cord stimulation and rehabilitation in an individual with chronic complete L1 paraplegia due to a conus medullaris injury: motor and functional outcomes at 18 months. Spinal Cord Ser Cases 2020;6(1):96.

56. Formento E, Minassian K, Wagner F, et al. Electrical spinal cord stimulation must preserve proprioception to enable locomotion in humans with spinal cord injury. Nat Neurosci 2018;21(12):1728–41.

57. Wagner FB, Mignardot JB, Le Goff-Mignardot CG, et al. Targeted neurotechnology restores walking in humans with spinal cord injury. Nature 2018; 563(7729):65–71.

58. Megia Garcia A, Serrano-Munoz D, Taylor J, et al. Transcutaneous spinal cord stimulation and motor rehabilitation in spinal cord injury: a systematic review. Neurorehabil Neural Repair 2020;34(1):3–12.

59. Minassian K, Persy I, Rattay F, et al. Posterior root-muscle reflexes elicited by transcutaneous stimulation of the human lumbosacral cord. Muscle Nerve 2007;35(3):327–36.

60. Inanici F, Samejima S, Gad P, et al. Transcutaneous electrical spinal stimulation promotes long-term recovery of upper extremity function in chronic tetraplegia. IEEE Trans Neural Syst Rehabil Eng 2018; 26(6):1272–8.

61. Gerasimenko YP, Lu DC, Modaber M, et al. Noninvasive reactivation of motor descending control after paralysis. J Neurotrauma 2015;32(24):1968–80.

62. Gad P, Lee S, Terrafranca N, et al. Non-invasive activation of cervical spinal networks after severe paralysis. J Neurotrauma 2018;35(18):2145–58.

63. Dimitrijevic MR, Dimitrijevic MM, Faganel J, et al. Suprasegmentally induced motor unit activity in paralyzed muscles of patients with established spinal cord injury. Ann Neurol 1984;16(2):216–21.

64. Sherwood AM, Dimitrijevic MR, McKay WB. Evidence of subclinical brain influence in clinically complete spinal cord injury: discomplete SCI. J Neurol Sci 1992;110(1–2):90–8.

65. Heald E, Hart R, Kilgore K, et al. Characterization of volitional electromyographic signals in the lower extremity after motor complete spinal cord injury. Neurorehabil Neural Repair 2017;31(6):583–91.

66. Kirshblum S, Millis S, McKinley W, et al. Late neurologic recovery after traumatic spinal cord injury. Arch Phys Med Rehabil 2004;85(11):1811–7.

67. Di Lazzaro V, Profice P, Ranieri F, et al. I-wave origin and modulation. Brain Stimul 2012;5(4):512–25.

68. D'Ostilio K, Goetz SM, Hannah R, et al. Effect of coil orientation on strength-duration time constant and I-wave activation with controllable pulse parameter transcranial magnetic stimulation. Clin Neurophysiol 2016;127(1):675–83.

69. Jo HJ, Di Lazzaro V, Perez MA. Effect of coil orientation on motor-evoked potentials in humans with tetraplegia. J Physiol 2018;596(20):4909–21.

70. Sriraman A, Oishi T, Madhavan S. Timing-dependent priming effects of tDCS on ankle motor skill learning. Brain Res 2014;1581:23–9.

71. Gomes-Osman J, Field-Fote EC. Improvements in hand function in adults with chronic tetraplegia following a multiday 10-Hz repetitive transcranial magnetic stimulation intervention combined with repetitive task practice. J Neurol Phys Ther 2015; 39(1):23–30.

72. Bunday KL, Perez MA. Motor recovery after spinal cord injury enhanced by strengthening corticospinal synaptic transmission. Curr Biol 2012;22(24): 2355–61.

73. Kumru H, Benito-Penalva J, Valls-Sole J, et al. Placebo-controlled study of rTMS combined with Lokomat((R)) gait training for treatment in subjects with motor incomplete spinal cord injury. Exp Brain Res 2016;234(12):3447–55.

74. James ND, McMahon SB, Field-Fote EC, et al. Neuromodulation in the restoration of function after spinal cord injury. Lancet Neurol 2018;17(10):905–17.

75. Capogrosso M, Milekovic T, Borton D, et al. A brain-spine interface alleviating gait deficits after spinal cord injury in primates. Nature 2016; 539(7628):284–8.

76. Musselman KE, Shah M, Zariffa J. Rehabilitation technologies and interventions for individuals with spinal cord injury: translational potential of current trends. J Neuroeng Rehabil 2018;15(1):40.

77. Querry RG, Pacheco F, Annaswamy T, et al. Synchronous stimulation and monitoring of soleus H reflex during robotic body weight-supported ambulation in subjects with spinal cord injury. J Rehabil Res Dev 2008;45(1):175–86.

78. Behrman AL, Lawless-Dixon AR, Davis SB, et al. Locomotor training progression and outcomes after incomplete spinal cord injury. Phys Ther 2005; 85(12):1356–71.

79. Griffin L, Decker MJ, Hwang JY, et al. Functional electrical stimulation cycling improves body composition, metabolic and neural factors in persons with spinal cord injury. J Electromyogr Kinesiol 2009;19(4):614–22.

80. van der Salm A, Veltink PH, Ijzerman MJ, et al. Comparison of electric stimulation methods for reduction of triceps surae spasticity in spinal cord injury. Arch Phys Med Rehabil 2006;87(2):222–8.

81. Martin R, Sadowsky C, Obst K, et al. Functional electrical stimulation in spinal cord injury: from theory to practice. Top Spinal Cord Inj Rehabil 2012;18(1):28–33.

82. Postans NJ, Hasler JP, Granat MH, et al. Functional electric stimulation to augment partial weight-bearing supported treadmill training for patients with acute incomplete spinal cord injury: a pilot study. Arch Phys Med Rehabil 2004;85(4):604–10.

83. Frotzler A, Coupaud S, Perret C, et al. Effect of detraining on bone and muscle tissue in subjects with chronic spinal cord injury after a period of electrically-stimulated cycling: a small cohort study. J Rehabil Med 2009;41(4):282–5.

84. Jeon JY, Weiss CB, Steadward RD, et al. Improved glucose tolerance and insulin sensitivity after electrical stimulation-assisted cycling in people with spinal cord injury. Spinal Cord 2002;40(3):110–7.

85. Scremin AM, Kurta L, Gentili A, et al. Increasing muscle mass in spinal cord injured persons with a functional electrical stimulation exercise program. Arch Phys Med Rehabil 1999;80(12):1531–6.

86. Sadowsky CL, McDonald JW. Activity-based restorative therapies: concepts and applications in spinal cord injury-related neurorehabilitation. Dev Disabil Res Rev 2009;15(2):112–6.

87. Barbeau H, Rossignol S. Recovery of locomotion after chronic spinalization in the adult cat. Brain Res 1987;412(1):84–95.

88. De Leon RD, Hodgson JA, Roy RR, et al. Full weight-bearing hindlimb standing following stand training in the adult spinal cat. J Neurophysiol 1998;80(1):83–91.

89. Grillner S, Rossignol S. On the initiation of the swing phase of locomotion in chronic spinal cats. Brain Res 1978;146(2):269–77.

90. Grillner S, Wallen P. Central pattern generators for locomotion, with special reference to vertebrates. Annu Rev Neurosci 1985;8:233–61.

91. Grillner S, Zangger P. On the central generation of locomotion in the low spinal cat. Exp Brain Res 1979;34(2):241–61.

92. Harkema SJ, Hurley SL, Patel UK, et al. Human lumbosacral spinal cord interprets loading during stepping. J Neurophysiol 1997;77(2):797–811.

93. Lovely RG, Gregor RJ, Roy RR, et al. Effects of training on the recovery of full-weight-bearing stepping in the adult spinal cat. Exp Neurol 1986;92(2): 421–35.

94. Hubli M, Dietz V. The physiological basis of neuro-rehabilitation–locomotor training after spinal cord injury. J Neuroeng Rehabil 2013;10:5.

95. Dietz V, Colombo G, Jensen L. Locomotor activity in spinal man. Lancet 1994;344(8932):1260–3.

96. Harkema SJ. Plasticity of interneuronal networks of the functionally isolated human spinal cord. Brain Res Rev 2008;57(1):255–64.

97. Castro MJ, Apple DF Jr, Hillegass EA, et al. Influence of complete spinal cord injury on skeletal muscle cross-sectional area within the first 6 months of injury. Eur J Appl Physiol Occup Physiol 1999;80(4):373–8.

98. Castro MJ, Apple DF Jr, Staron RS, et al. Influence of complete spinal cord injury on skeletal muscle within 6 mo of injury. J Appl Physiol (1985) 1999; 86(1):350–8.

99. Massucci M, Brunetti G, Piperno R, et al. Walking with the advanced reciprocating gait orthosis (ARGO) in thoracic paraplegic patients: energy expenditure and cardiorespiratory performance. Spinal Cord 1998;36(4):223–7.

100. Cheung EYY, Yu KKK, Kwan RLC, et al. Effect of EMG-biofeedback robotic-assisted body weight supported treadmill training on walking ability and cardiopulmonary function on people with subacute spinal cord injuries - a randomized controlled trial. BMC Neurol 2019;19(1):140.

101. Sale P, Franceschini M, Waldner A, et al. Use of the robot assisted gait therapy in rehabilitation of patients with stroke and spinal cord injury. Eur J Phys Rehabil Med 2012;48(1):111–21.

102. Aach M, Cruciger O, Sczesny-Kaiser M, et al. Voluntary driven exoskeleton as a new tool for rehabilitation in chronic spinal cord injury: a pilot study. Spine J 2014;14(12):2847–53.

103. Cruciger O, Tegenthoff M, Schwenkreis P, et al. Locomotion training using voluntary driven exoskeleton (HAL) in acute incomplete. SCI *Neurol* 2014;83(5):474.

104. Baunsgaard CB, Nissen UV, Brust AK, et al. Exoskeleton gait training after spinal cord injury: an exploratory study on secondary health conditions. J Rehabil Med 2018;50(9):806–13.

105. Nam KY, Kim HJ, Kwon BS, et al. Robot-assisted gait training (Lokomat) improves walking function and activity in people with spinal cord injury: a systematic review. J Neuroeng Rehabil 2017; 14(1):24.

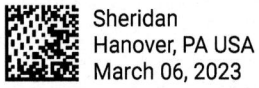